CREATIVE SPA

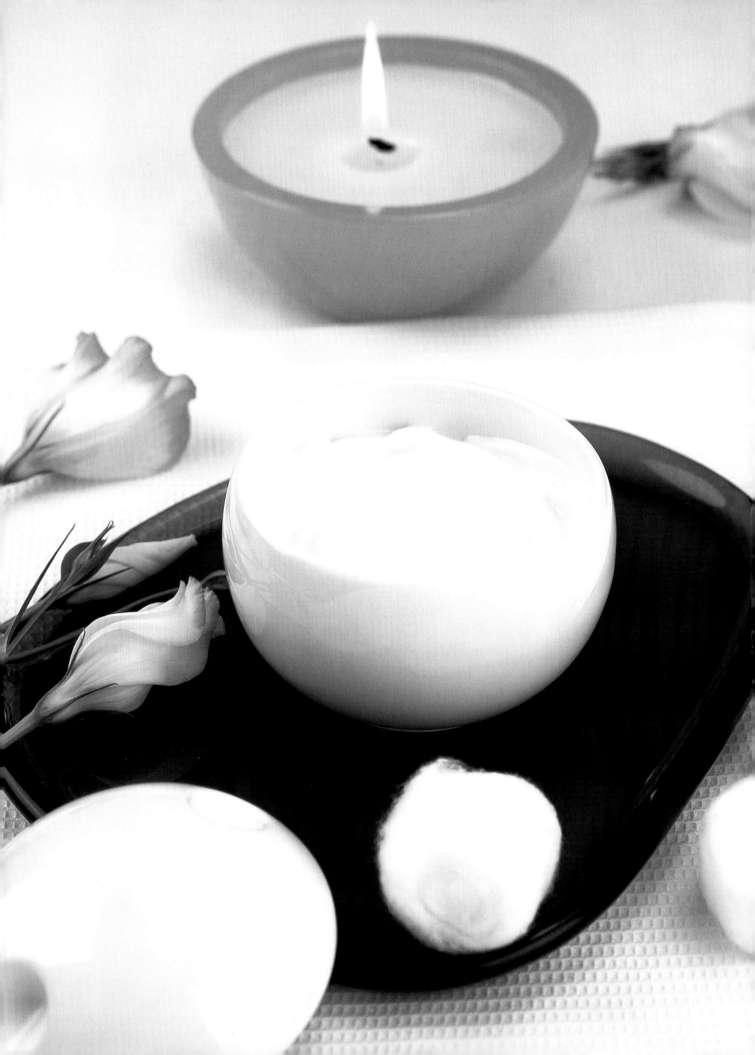

CREATIVE SPA

MAKE YOUR OWN SKIN CARE PRODUCTS

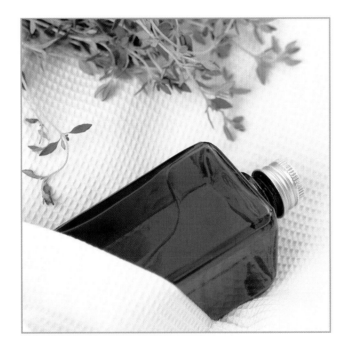

Cheryl Coutts and Ada Warren

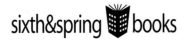

FOR ANDREW

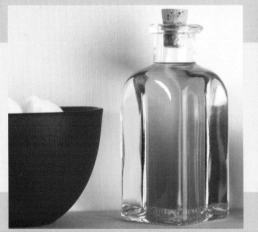
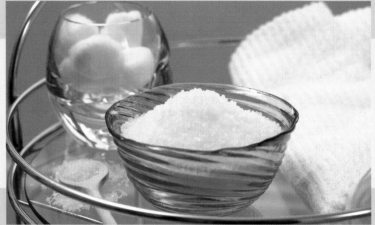

© New Holland Publishers (UK) Ltd

First published in 2005 in the USA by

Sixth&Spring Books
An Imprint of Soho Publishing Company
233 Spring St., 8th floor
New York, NY 10013

First published in 2004 in the UK by
New Holland Publishers (UK) Ltd
Garfield House, 86–88 Edgware Road, London W2 2EA, United Kingdom
www.newhollandpublishers.com

Library of Congress Control Number: 2004116752

ISBN 1-931543-76-3

Senior Editor: Clare Sayer
Design: Isobel Gillan
Production: Hazel Kirkman
Photographer: Shona Wood
Editorial Direction: Rosemary Wilkinson
Cover design: Chi Ling Moy

Manufactured in Malaysia

1 3 5 7 9 10 8 6 4 2

CONTENTS

INTRODUCTION

Life is often hectic and tiring; stress is never far away. We should all make time for special treats, and the bathroom is the perfect place to start. Bath time can be a great "switch-off-and-relax time," an opportunity to pamper body and soul. It was with this daily wind-down in mind that we began making our own soaps, because we couldn't find commercial products that moisturized our skin the way we wanted and smelled exquisite. Making your own soap and other items for the bath and spa—including creams, shampoos, massage oils, and shave lotions—allows you to use natural ingredients, such as essential oils, to achieve an overall feeling of well-being, as well as pamper the skin and senses. In this book, we have collected a number of our favorite recipes for you to try for yourself.

This book features recipes for all times of the day and all members of the family. There are treats for the shower, because there is nothing better than a morning boost to leave you delicately fragranced and ready to meet the world head-on, while our night creams will work their magic while you sleep. There are shampoos for the children and plenty of soaps, creams, and shave products for the men in your clan. There are lotions to use from top to toe, and even recipes that target specific complaints, such as varicose veins or sunburn.

What's more, none of these recipes will leave you smelling like you've been sprayed by every perfume seller on the ground floor of a department store. This is because essential oils, which are used to fragrance and lend distinction to each recipe, have gentle, natural aromas that will soothe you and those around you.

We both love growing our own fresh herbs, which we use in our soapmaking as well as in our cooking. We make soap for the same reason that we cook—because we love it—and our friends and family are willing guinea pigs for all our new inventions. We hope that you will have as much fun as we do as you work your way through this book. None of the recipes is difficult, so don't be scared to try them all. And once you get the hang of the various processes and the qualities of each essential oil, you can adapt our recipes to suit your own tastes and needs.

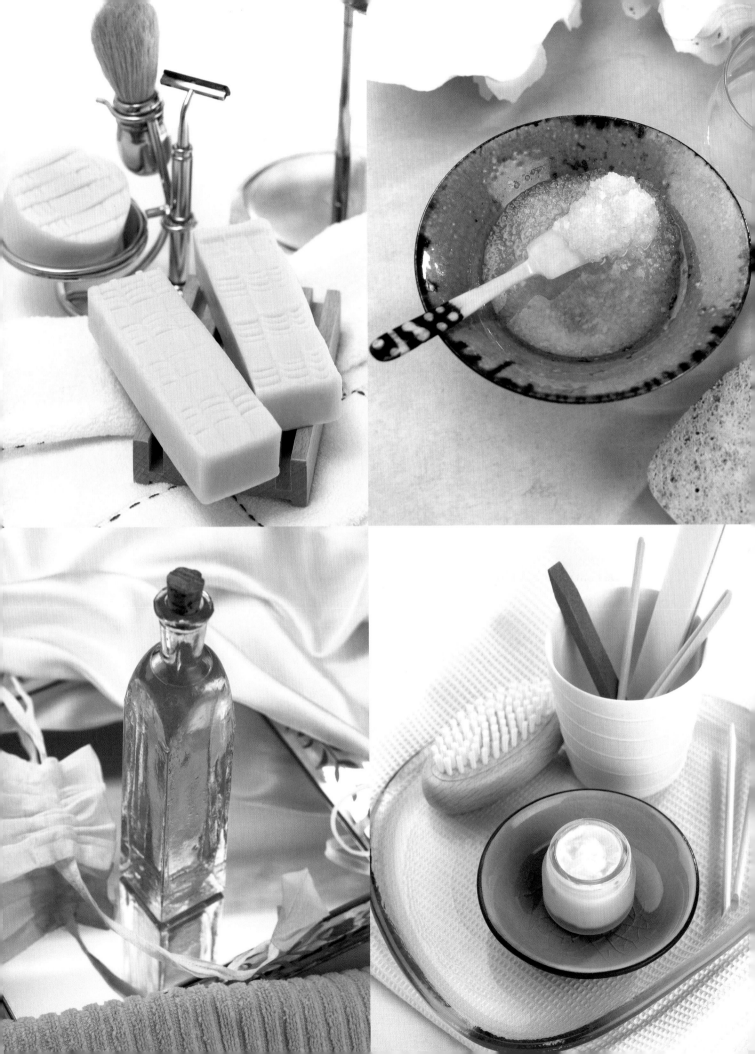

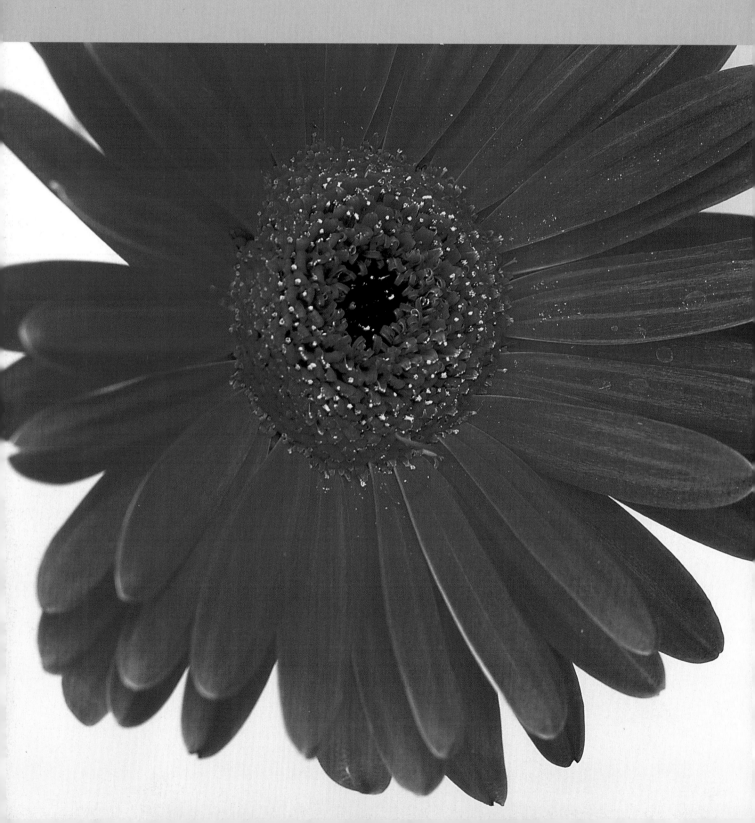

BASIC INFORMATION

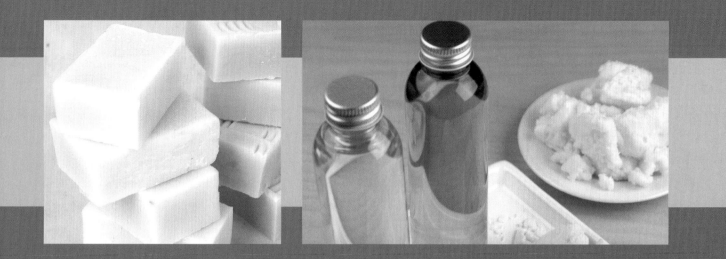

A HISTORY OF SOAP AND BATHING

The origins of personal cleanliness date back to prehistoric times. Since water is essential for life, the earliest people lived near water and knew something about its cleansing properties—at least that it was useful for rinsing the mud off their hands.

A soaplike material found in clay cylinders during the excavation of ancient Babylon is evidence that soapmaking was known as early as 2800 BC. Inscriptions on the cylinders suggest that fats were boiled with ashes to make soap. Records also show that ancient Egyptians bathed regularly. The Ebers papyrus, a medical document from about 1500 BC, describes the process of mixing animal fats, vegetable oils, and alkaline salts to form a soap, used for washing and treating skin diseases.

The early Greeks bathed for aesthetic reasons and apparently did not use soap. Instead, they cleaned their bodies with blocks of clay, sand, pumice, and ashes, then anointed themselves with oil and scraped off the oil and dirt with a metal instrument known as a *strigil*.

As Roman civilization advanced, so did bathing. The first of the Roman baths, supplied with water from aqueducts, was built in about 312 BC. The baths were luxurious, and bathing became very popular. Soap

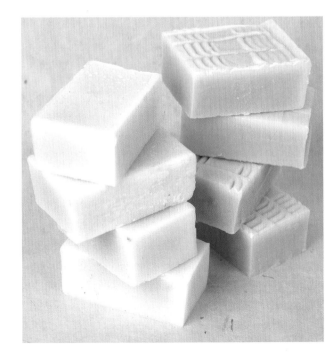

acquired its name, according to Roman legend, from Mount Sapo, where animals were sacrificed. Rain washed a mixture of melted animal fat and wood ashes down into the clay soil along the Tiber River. Women found that this mixture cleaned their washing with less effort.

After the fall of Rome in AD 467, and the resulting decline in bathing habits, much of Europe felt the impact of filth upon public health. The lack of personal cleanliness contributed heavily to the great plagues of the Middle Ages, and it wasn't until the 17th century that bathing started to come back into fashion in much of Europe. However, in other parts of the medieval world, personal cleanliness remained important. Daily bathing was a common custom in Japan during the Middle Ages, and in Iceland pools warmed with water from hot springs were popular gathering places.

Soapmaking was an established craft in Europe by the 7th century. Soapmaking guilds guarded their trade secrets closely. Gradually more varieties of soap became available for shaving and shampooing, bathing and laundering. Italy, Spain, and France were early centers of soap manufacturing, owing to the ready supply of raw materials such as olive oil. The English began making soap during the 12th century. For many years soapmaking remained, essentially, a household chore. Eventually, professional soapmakers began collecting waste fats from households, in exchange for some soap. A major step toward large-scale commercial soapmaking occurred in 1791 when a French chemist, Nicholas Leblanc, patented a process for making soda ash from common salt. Soda ash, also known as sodium carbonate or caustic soda, is the alkali obtained from ashes that combines with fat to form soap. The Leblanc process yielded quantities of good-quality, inexpensive soda ash.

Well into the 19th century, soap was heavily taxed as a luxury item by many countries. When the high tax was removed, soap became available to ordinary people and cleanliness standards improved throughout the world.

Scientific discoveries over the past 200 years have made soapmaking one of the world's fastest-growing industries. At the same time, its broad availability changed soap from a luxury item to an everyday necessity.

PRINCIPLES OF SOAPMAKING

Making soap is really quite easy and can be lots of fun. Quite simply, soap is created when an oil or combination of oils (which are usually acid) is mixed with an alkaline solution of sodium hydroxide (caustic soda) and water, otherwise known as lye water. The chemical reaction that occurs is known as "saponification," which occurs in stages in what is known as the "cold process" method. This is the science behind the process. You will find detailed instructions in each recipe or in the basic techniques section on page 18.

Weighing and measuring
The recipes in this book list the exact amount of ingredients to use, including oils, caustic soda, and mineral water. The correct proportion of oil to lye water is a crucial factor in the soapmaking process.

Saponification
This is the chemical process that occurs when the oils and lye water are mixed. During the curing process (see below), the alkali in the lye water is neutralized, so although soap is made with sodium hydroxide (caustic soda), once cured it does not contain it.

pH balance
This is the measure of the acidity or alkalinity of a substance. The skin is slightly acid at a pH of 5.5, and most cold-process soaps are between pH 8 and 9. This can be measured using litmus paper. Any soap reading above pH 10 should be discarded, because it is too alkaline. Some commercial soaps have their alkalinity reduced artificially to make them "neutral," but the chemicals used to do this probably make the soaps worse to wash with than a more alkaline soap.

Tracing
Tracing is the term used to describe the point at which the base mixture has been stirred and thickened adequately. When a little of the soap drizzled over the surface of the mixture leaves a line or "trace," you can proceed with adding essential oils, herbs, or seeds to the soap.

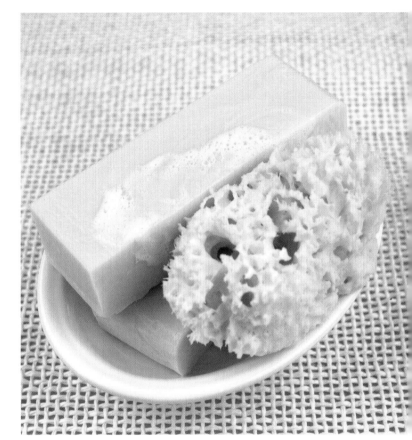

Setting
After being poured into the mold, the soap needs to be left to set. Cover with a sheet of cardboard and leave in a warm, dry place. Setting times can vary from soap to soap and depend on a number of factors, such as room temperature and ingredients used. As a basic guide, your soap should be solid enough to remove from the mold 24 to 48 hours after you have poured it. It should be easy enough to cut the soap into bars at this stage.

Curing or maturation
Once the soap has been turned out and cut, it must be allowed to mature for at least four weeks before being used. Any residual sodium hydroxide (lye) is neutralized during this time. Sometimes, this can result in changes to the appearance of your soap, such as a fine white dust on the surface of the soap (see page 21). Turn the soaps regularly to equalize their drying rates.

EQUIPMENT

GENERAL EQUIPMENT

Most of the equipment you need to make the projects in this book can be found in your kitchen cupboards. However, it is probably a good idea to keep a few basic utensils, such as a saucepan and some bowls, set aside especially for soapmaking.

Bowls Make sure you have a few measuring bowls on hand for weighing caustic soda and solid oils. Plastic bowls will not be corroded by caustic soda.

Cardboard Sheets of cardboard are used to cover a mold of soap while it sets overnight. You can also use heavy cardboard sheets as cutting boards.

Carving knife You will need a sharp knife to cut your soap into bars. Cookie cutters can also be used to make novel shapes.

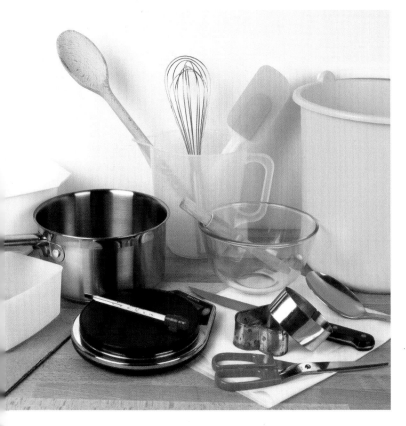

Dark-colored or opaque containers with lids Creams and massage oils are transferred to glass jars or bottles with lids for storage. Dark-colored or opaque jars are particularly useful because they protect the essential oils in the mix from exposure to light.

Jam thermometers Jam thermometers are perfect for measuring the temperature of the oils and lye water during soapmaking. It is a good idea to have three thermometers: one for oils, one for lye water, and a spare.

Kitchen scales Accurate scales are a necessity when soapmaking. Modern versions are preferable, because you will need to measure some ingredients in small amounts of less than an ounce.

Measuring cups It is useful to have two measuring cups—one for oil, one for water. Plastic or Pyrex kinds should be used, because metal ones will corrode.

Pastry brush Use this to oil the plastic soap mold.

Plastic molds You can buy special soap molds, but plastic containers work just as well.

Plastic spatula A plastic spatula will not corrode when used to stir the lye water and the soap mix. You can use a wooden spoon, but it will not last as long.

Spoons Stainless-steel spoons can be used to mix the heated oils when making soap. A wooden spoon is used to beat the water and oils together when making creams.

Stainless-steel saucepan Use a heavy-bottomed stainless-steel saucepan for melting the oils. A double boiler is not essential for basic soapmaking.

Stainless-steel whisk A large stainless-steel whisk can be used to whisk creams and mix soap until tracing occurs.

Tall plastic bucket The bucket in which you dilute the caustic soda must be plastic, because metal ones will corrode. A tall bucket is safest, since there is less chance of the lye water splashing out.

Waxed paper and scissors You will need to line plastic soap molds with waxed paper, which is simply cut with scissors.

SAFETY EQUIPMENT
The only potentially dangerous processes of soapmaking are handling the caustic soda, the lye water, and the raw soap before it has matured, and perhaps using the carving knife to cut it. The following items are necessary to protect you and your clothes.

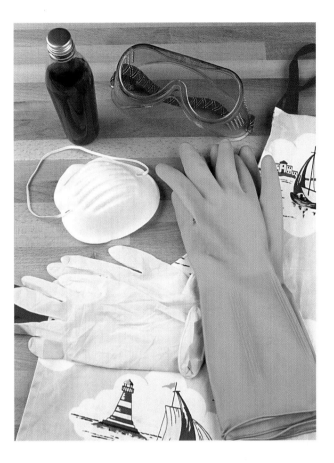

Apron A heavy-duty apron is useful for shielding your clothes from splashes and spills.

Face mask When caustic soda is mixed with water, potentially harmful fumes rise from the bowl. Wear a mask to stop you from breathing them in.

Gloves Protecting your hands is particularly important when handling caustic soda or lye water. At this stage, wear rubber gloves. We wear long ones over long-sleeved tops. Latex gloves are useful when you are cutting and turning the soap, because at this stage you need to be more gentle with it, but remember that it is still caustic until completely cured.

Safety goggles Always wear eye protection during soapmaking and cleaning. Protective goggles can be bought in home-improvement and hardware stores.

Vinegar Always keep a bottle of vinegar on hand when making soap, because in the event of the caustic mixture spilling or splashing onto your skin, rinsing with vinegar will neutralize the alkali. Rinse off with water.

Safety first
While soapmaking is relatively easy and fun to do, it does involve caustic substances, high temperatures, and chemical reactions. The following safety considerations should always be followed:

- Wear protective clothing: goggles, a face mask, an apron, and long rubber gloves.
- Caustic soda should not be ingested. If it is, go to the nearest hospital immediately.
- Always wear goggles when handling caustic material. Splashes on the skin are painful, and splashes in your eyes could be devastating. If caustic soda is splashed into the eyes, rinse with cold water and rush to see a doctor.
- Splashes on the skin at any point during the soapmaking process should be rinsed with vinegar, then water.
- Store caustic soda in an airtight container and label it clearly. Keep it out of the reach of children and pets.
- Do not allow children or pets anywhere near the soapmaking process.
- Keep soapmaking utensils separate from other kitchen utensils.
- Scrape the remains of the soap from the saucepan carefully (wearing rubber gloves) into a bag, seal, and then place in the garbage.
- Carefully wash all the utensils.
- Never leave soap pans unattended. Better to make soap with a friend, anyway!

INGREDIENTS

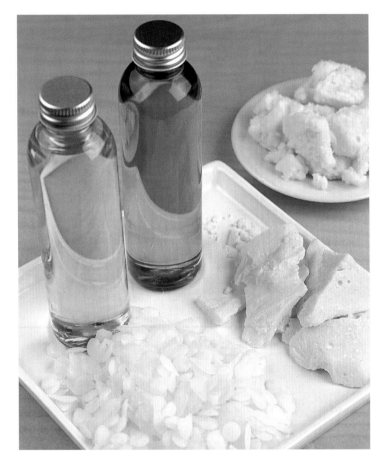

Avocado oil High in vitamins A, D, and E, avocado oil is excellent for mature, cracked skin. It revitalizes, heals, and regenerates cells.

Beeswax Beeswax is used in the process of making soaps and creams. It can be used in its natural form (yellow beeswax), but bear in mind that this will color the soap. We use bleached beeswax, which gives the whiteness to our soap recipes. Beeswax thickens other oils to a suitable consistency in creams.

Calendula oil A mildly antiseptic oil that is cleansing, soothing, and healing. This oil softens and smoothes skin.

Cocoa butter Cocoa butter attracts and holds moisture to the skin, thus softening it.

Coconut oil This oil comes as a solid and is wonderfully moisturizing. It also makes soap lather.

Evening primrose oil This lovely oil helps prevent premature aging of the skin.

Olive oil Olive oil prevents loss of natural moisture, as well as softens the skin and attracts external moisture to it.

Palm oil This is another product from the coconut palm and, like coconut oil, it is solid. However, it is slightly creamier and has a softer texture.

Pomace oil This oil is produced from the second and third pressings of the olive. It is slightly less expensive than extra-virgin olive oil.

Rosehip oil A natural preservative, this is sometimes used in shampoos.

Sunflower oil A conditioning oil that stabilizes lather.

Sweet almond oil Sweet almond is a conditioning, emollient oil that softens and smoothes the skin.

All the basic ingredients for our recipes are readily available from hardware stores, supermarkets, and drug stores, while whole-foods stores are a good place to stock up on herbs. Asian supermarkets will provide coconut oil and palm oil if your normal supermarket does not stock them.

BASE OILS

Many different oils can be used as the base of a soap, massage oil, or cream. When making soaps, we tend to combine emollient oils—such as olive, coconut, sweet almond, and avocado oils—with palm oil, which helps to make a harder soap. As you gain confidence with soapmaking, you may decide to experiment with other oils and combinations of oils. If so, you may need to vary the amount of lye water you use, because different oils have different saponification rates.

Vitamin E oil This is a good oil for preventing wrinkles.

Wheat germ oil This is exceptional for facial soaps because it is particularly gentle.

THE OTHER ESSENTIALS

The following ingredients form an essential part of the recipes and can be found in large supermarkets or health-food shops.

Caustic soda Otherwise known as sodium hydroxide, this is the alkali that is combined with the acidic oils to make soap. Because it is caustic, the set soap needs to cure for at least four weeks, until the sodium hydroxide is neutralized. Caustic soda can be found in hardware or home-improvement stores. Make sure the caustic soda you buy is at least 95 percent pure.

Dead Sea salt This is used to make bath salts and exfoliating scrubs. It is important to use Dead Sea salt, which is purer than any other. Maldon sea salt flakes can also be used; they are slightly less abrasive.

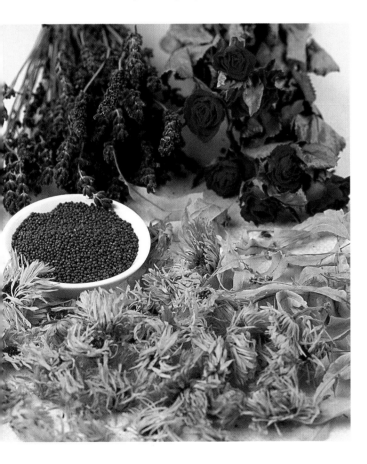

Glycerine This clear, syrupy liquid can be added to soap to increase its moisturizing properties. It is available at pharmacies.

Mineral water Water is a crucial ingredient in soapmaking. Its main job is to dissolve the caustic soda to create lye water. Pure water is best, so mineral water and bottled distilled water are good options.

Vodka We use vodka in some of our recipes because it is the purest form of alcohol. It is a great toner and pore cleanser.

Witch hazel This clear, slightly astringent liquid is available at pharmacies.

ADDITIVES AND EXTRAS

The following ingredients are designed to give your soap or bath product its delicious aroma and wonderful texture. They are what make your homemade spa product such a treat.

Dried flowers and seeds Dried flower petals make a good addition to soaps because they give the soap a pretty, speckled appearance and can have a slightly exfoliating effect. Calendula and chamomile are good examples. We often add mustard seeds to give soap a wonderful means of exfoliating. Dried herbs can also be used in the same way.

Essential oils Essentials oils not only give your homemade bath products the most wonderful scent, they also have properties that affect your health and mood. See pages 16 and 17 for a glossary of essential oils and their properties. Essential oils can be bought at most drug or vitamin stores, and the price of each oil will vary. Essential oils are very potent and used only in small amounts, specified by number of drops. Keep essential oils in a cool, dark place in jars with tight-fitting lids. Use only pure oils.

Seaweed Seaweed is a great product for improving the texture of the skin. You can buy seaweed in powdered form from health-food stores. We like to use Japanese arame seaweed, which has a nice texture and great therapeutic qualities.

GLOSSARY OF ESSENTIAL OILS

Each essential oil has sensual and mood-enhancing properties, and can help to soothe particular ailments.

Bay An uplifting oil ideal for helping to stimulate memory, concentration, and confidence. Also good for stomach complaints and aches and pains, and for easing cold and flu symptoms.

Benzoin A beautiful, warm, vanilla-like oil. Its sedative effects make it ideal for dealing with sleep problems, anxiety, and grief. Also excellent for helping relieve breathing difficulties, asthma, coughs, colds, and chills.

Bergamot This citrus oil, produced from orange rind, is a refreshing, uplifting oil, good for alleviating anxiety and stress.

Black pepper A stimulating oil that helps strengthen the nerves and mind, as well as warm muscles, making it useful in easing the discomfort of arthritis, muscle pains, and sprains.

Cedarwood This is a wonderful tonic to the skin, especially if it is dry or cracked. It can be used to ease coughs, especially the dry, persistent type. When used with citrus oils, it may lift depression, soothe nerves, and ease stress. This deeply relaxing oil is also an aphrodisiac, as popular with men as with women.

Chamomile, Roman This sedative oil is ideal for soothing pain of any sort and is particularly effective in children. It helps with anxiety, sleep problems, and anger, plus arthritis, headache, migraine, and stomach problems.

Cinnamon Warming and antiseptic, it stimulates and relaxes, giving it a reputation as a mild aphrodisiac.

Clary sage A sedative oil that is ideal for those who find it difficult to "switch off." Also excellent for treating premenstrual tension and menstrual cramps, as well as muscle pain, labor pain, and night sweats. It is also a good skin conditioner.

Eucalyptus An oil to revive the spirit and ease cough and cold symptoms, muscular pain, and arthritis. Eucalyptus boosts immunity and can ease headaches, sinusitis, and insect bites, as well as repel insects.

Frankincense A sedative oil ideal for addressing sleep problems and anxiety, helping produce feelings of inner peace and acceptance. Useful in treating coughs and asthma, and a great addition to face creams for dry or mature skin.

Geranium An uplifting oil ideal for helping ease mood swings, postnatal depression, and premenstrual tension. It is used frequently in beauty care because it is good for most skin types. It is also an excellent mosquito repellent.

Ginger A stimulating, warm oil ideal for treating muscle pain, arthritic joint problems, sprains, and strains. It eases coughs and colds and boosts immunity, as well as easing stomach problems such as sickness, travel sickness, and nausea.

Grapefruit A refreshing and reviving oil with euphoric qualities. It is great to use for oily skin and excellent for remedying the blues and exhaustion.

Juniper berry This oil is known for its detoxification properties, which is why it is used to treat arthritis, hangovers, water retention, and cellulite, and to clear emotional "baggage" that stops you from moving on in life. Invaluable!

Lavender What can't this oil do? It can be used to ease burns, sunburn, arthritis, and any "hot" conditions because of its cooling effects. It can help alleviate eczema, acne, insect bites, stings, head lice, bruises, headaches, vertigo, migraines, fainting, aches, pains, and sprains.

Lemon Ideal for treating cold sores, warts, and athlete's foot. A very uplifting detox oil that is used for cellulite, gout, arthritis, colds, flu, and infection, and to help reduce nightmares when mixed with a suitable sedative oil. Children respond especially well to it.

Lemongrass An uplifting, refreshing oil that can be used to treat excessive perspiration, athlete's foot, muscle pain, poor circulation, and head lice, and to help improve muscle tone.

Lime An uplifting member of the citrus-oil family with a mouthwatering aroma.

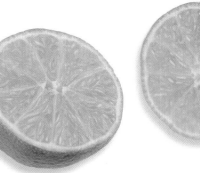

Mandarin An uplifting oil that smells good enough to eat, so it is no surprise that it is used to treat stomach problems and depression. Children love it and an anxious child responds well to having a diluted mixture rubbed clockwise into the tummy. Also used to reduce stretch marks and scarring, reduce premenstrual tension, and increase appetite, especially following illness.

May chang This uplifting oil is great for helping ease depression and keeping away the winter blues.

Myrrh Myrrh is a deep-smelling oil with a warm, woody aroma, useful for dealing with sorrow, anger, rejection, and promoting feelings of tranquillity. It is also excellent for treating athlete's foot and other fungal infections; soothing asthma, coughs, gum infections, and thrush; and boosting immunity. A very powerful antiseptic.

Patchouli An excellent tonic for the skin, patchouli can be used to treat athlete's foot, acne, dandruff, and eczema. It is also an insect repellent and has been used as an aphrodisiac. It can ease depression and, in small doses, lethargy.

Peppermint This stimulating oil can be used to ease headaches and migraines if used at the onset of an attack. It can aid memory and reduce fatigue. It also warms muscles and eases pains, colds, coughs, and flu. It can also help colic and stomach cramps, as well as fainting.

Petitgrain This oil is widely used for combating the winter blues. It is ideal for convalescence, nervous exhaustion, mild depression, nervousness, and self-blame. It is also used to treat acne and oily skin.

Rosemary This potent pick is as useful and versatile as lavender in that it can treat dandruff, lice, varicose veins, and scabies, as well as muscle pains, arthritis, rheumatism, cellulite, poor circulation, digestion problems, bronchitis, whooping cough, coughs, colds, flu, headaches, poor memory, and more.

Sage Used in very small amounts, this oil is soothing and antiseptic, excellent for joints and muscles. Reduces sweatiness.

Sweet orange An uplifting oil that is good for tension and depression—and for people who find it hard to "switch off."

Tangerine A light, happy citrus oil with uplifting, freshening properties.

Tea tree Well-known for its antiseptic, antiviral, and antibacterial properties, tea tree is also good for combating certain fungal infections, sinusitis, chest infections, mouth ulcers, athlete's foot, blemishes, boils, insect bites, cystitis, and thrush. It is good for convalescence, even after shock.

Thyme This distinctively fragranced oil can treat colds, coughs, and flu and ease headaches, pain, sciatica, and sprains.

Ylang ylang This floral exotic oil has been used widely to ease stress, depression, fear, anger (especially if it is born of frustration), high blood pressure, shock, panic attacks, and palpitations. It is also useful for general skin care and is an aphrodisiac to boot. Lovely mixed with citrus oils to make it lighter and more refreshing.

Safety with essential oils

Essential oils are highly concentrated. Although beneficial, their strength and effects should not be underestimated. In this book, we have suggested essential oils to be used in the recipes. These will be fine for most people, but if you have a particular health problem, are taking any medications, or are pregnant, you should seek professional medical advice before using any essential oils. Some essential oils can be harmful if used inappropriately.

- Do not apply undiluted essential oils directly to the skin, except lavender, which can be used in very small doses.
- Do not ingest the oils.
- Avoid contact with the eyes.
- If you have sensitive skin or allergies, consult a professional before using essential oils.
- Keep essential oils out of the reach of children.
- Avoid using citrus oils (bergamot, grapefruit, lemon, lime, mandarin, sweet orange, tangerine) for at least 12 hours before sunbathing or using a tanning bed.

THE BASIC TECHNIQUES

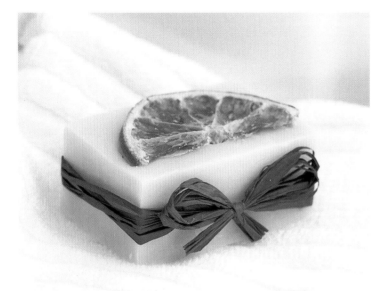

Each of the recipes in this book has a full set of instructions. However, you may find it useful to look at the following photographs and step-by-step instructions before you begin a recipe, to ensure that you are confident with the whole technique.

SOAPMAKING: THE COLD PROCESS METHOD

This book uses the cold process method of making soap, which is the most natural and does not involve the use of chemical additives. Commercial soap is often made using tallow (animal fat) and contains many synthetic perfumes, colors, and preservatives. For this reason, it can dry and irritate the skin. In fact, many people believe they are sensitive to all soaps, when in fact they would be perfectly fine using our gentle, natural, therapeutic bars. Follow our simple soapmaking instructions and experience the difference.

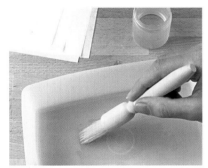

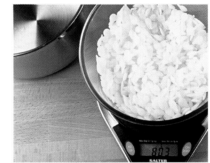

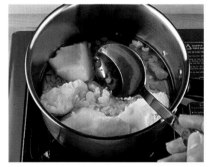

1 Use a pastry brush and a little sunflower oil to lightly grease a plastic mold. You can buy custom-made soap molds, but plastic food-storage containers and trays work just as well. Line the base and sides of the mold with waxed paper, tidying the corners and smoothing down well. Use more oil to "stick down" any loose bits of paper.

2 Measure the solid oils first, then place them in a stainless-steel sauce-pan with a heavy base. Measure the liquid oils and add these to the pan.

3 Heat the oils over low heat, stirring with a stainless-steel spoon or plastic spatula until the oils are combined.

Think ahead
Making soap is a bit like cooking—some people find it daunting at first. As with cooking, it is best to have all your ingredients and equipment ready at the start. Make sure that the base oils, lye water ingredients, essential oils, herbs, seeds, and petals are measured and at your fingertips, so that you don't find yourself searching for an ingredient at a crucial moment and ruining the process.

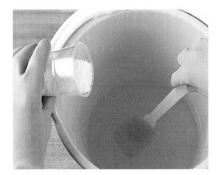 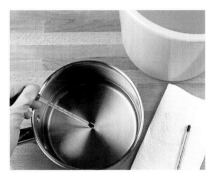 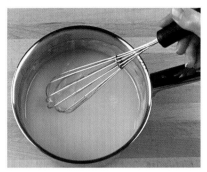

4 Make sure the room is well ventilated and wear goggles, a face mask, rubber gloves, and an apron. Measure the caustic soda in a plastic bowl and set aside. Pour a measured amount of mineral water into a tall plastic bucket. Carefully pour the caustic soda into the mineral water. Fumes will be given off at this stage. Stir with a plastic spatula until dissolved. The caustic mixture (lye water) will be very hot at this point.

5 Use a jam thermometer to test the temperature of the lye water as it cools. To help cool it, place the bucket in a sinkful of cold water and stir. When it nears the required temperature, reheat or cool the base oils as required. Both the lye water and the melted oils need to reach the same temperature of 131°F; you will need two thermometers to monitor this.

6 When both the oils and the lye water have reached the right temperature, remove the pan from the heat and pour the lye water into the oils. Stir thoroughly with a whisk and continue until tracing occurs. This is when the soap thickens and a spoonful of soap drizzled over the surface leaves a visible line. It can take 10 minutes or an hour, depending on the oils used. The soaps in this book will all trace within 20 minutes.

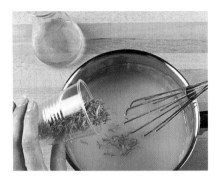 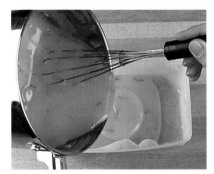 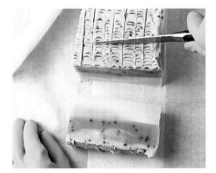

7 Add the essential oils, herbs, petals, or seeds at this stage, stirring thoroughly.

8 Pour the mixture into the prepared mold. Place in a safe, warm, and dry place. Cover the mold with cardboard and leave for 24 hours.

9 Wearing protective gloves, turn out the soap onto waxed paper. Use a carving knife to cut the soap into bars and lay them out on a tray covered with waxed paper, with room for air to circulate around them. Place in a warm, dry place to cure. Leave for four weeks, turning occasionally to dry all sides.

Alternatively, use cookie cutters to make shaped soaps. Simply press the cutter firmly and evenly into the soap after you have turned it out, and leave to cure as above.

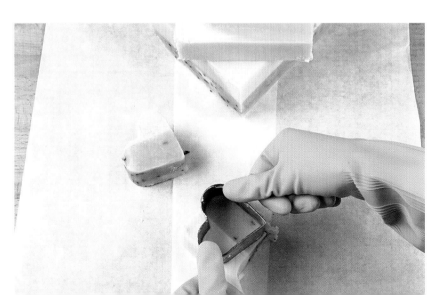

MAKING HERBAL INFUSIONS

Herbal infusions are used in a number of recipes in this book but they are also a great way to tone your skin, as well as being inexpensive. Simply infuse flowers such as calendula (pot marigold), lime, elder, or chamomile to make a very effective face splash. It will keep only for a few days, so apply liberally. It can be mixed with witch hazel in equal parts for a slightly astringent toner that is ideal for normal, combination, or oily skin.

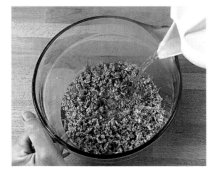

1 Place a double handful of flowers in a jug and pour over 1 pint of boiling water—although this is not an exact science. Cover and leave to cool.

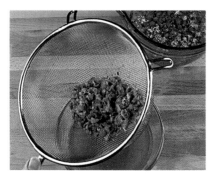

2 Strain the mixture and keep it in the fridge. It is incredibly refreshing and great for hair, too, if you really strain all the bits out.

MAKING SKIN CREAMS

There is no caustic material used in the making of creams, so no particular safety tips are applicable. Just take care as you would with cooking—wear an apron to protect clothes, and handle hot fats and water carefully. Our creams do not contain preservatives, so they should be made in small quantities and used within a month. Keep them refrigerated when possible or in a cool, dark place.

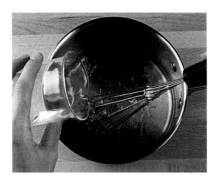

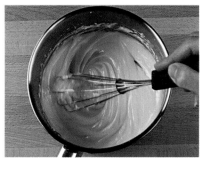

1 Measure the oils and place in a stainless-steel saucepan. Set over low heat and stir gently until all the oils have melted.

2 Measure the water and add to the oils in the pan, whisking or stirring with a wooden spoon until the mixture thickens and turns creamy.

3 Remove from the heat and stir until the cream has cooled to room temperature. Add the essential oils.

4 Transfer to glass jars with lids and shake gently until the cream has cooled, to stop the oil and water from separating.

MAKING OILS

Simple recipes such as the Wide-Awake Massage Oil on page 26 or the Thymeless Sleep Oil on page 78 do not require any complicated techniques. Simply measure the oils as directed and pour into a suitable container with a tight-fitting lid. Shake gently to mix.

MAKING SALTS AND SCRUBS

Salts and scrubs are easy to make and no caustic material is used. The salts should be used within two months.

1 Mix all the oils together, then stir in Dead Sea salt.

2 Transfer the salts to a dark glass jar with a lid.

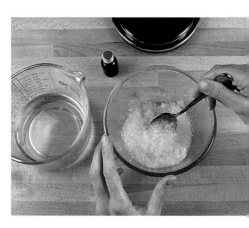

TROUBLESHOOTING

Don't worry, we all face glitches from time to time. Some can be overcome, while others may mean that you have to start all over again.

RELATIVELY MINOR PROBLEMS

These errors may result in a soap that is not as visually appealing as it should be but that can still be used.

Soft soap If the soap is too soft to cut, you may have used too little caustic soda or it was not pure (it should be 95 percent at least). Leave a little longer to dry, then try to cut it again; it may dry after a few more weeks.

Crumbly soap This soap has lost heat too rapidly or may have been combined at too low a temperature. It can be used but may not look as good as usual. Test the pH to be on the safe side.

White film A white film on the surface of the soap is nothing to worry about, just a little soda ash. Scrape it off to make the soap look more attractive.

Oil on the surface A little oil on the surface means that the soap may have been stirred too little. The oil may sink with time; otherwise, it can be wiped off when the soap is cut. Test for pH, because if too much oil is lost, the soap will be caustic.

No tracing Certain oils take longer to saponify, such as extra-virgin olive oil, so just keep stirring. If after one hour there is still no tracing, it may be due to the lye being poured into the oils at too low a temperature. Time to start again, we're afraid.

Seizing Occasionally the soap will suddenly thicken on the addition of certain essential oils, notably clove. This can be alarming, but don't worry. Just pour it immediately into the mold. If the surface won't flatten, make a nice pattern with a fork and knife, like icing a cake.

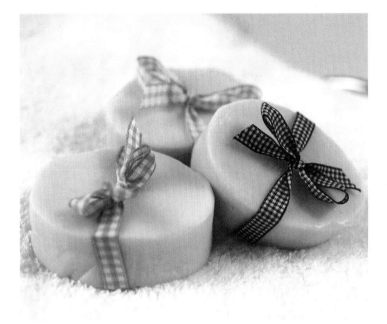

BIG TROUBLE: DISCARD THE SOAP

We're afraid there is no hope if your soap has any of these problems. Don't even think about using it.

Air pockets filled with liquid This problem is due to insufficient stirring, but, more importantly, the soap may be caustic and should not be used.

Thick layer of oil on the surface This problem is usually due to lack of stirring or a rapid temperature loss. If too much oil separates, then the soap will be too caustic and must be discarded.

Large amounts of white powder This is caused by too much caustic soda in the mix. It also means that the pH balance of the soap is too high, so the soap must be discarded.

Brittle soap Again, this occurs when there is too much caustic soda in the soap and means the soap will have to be discarded.

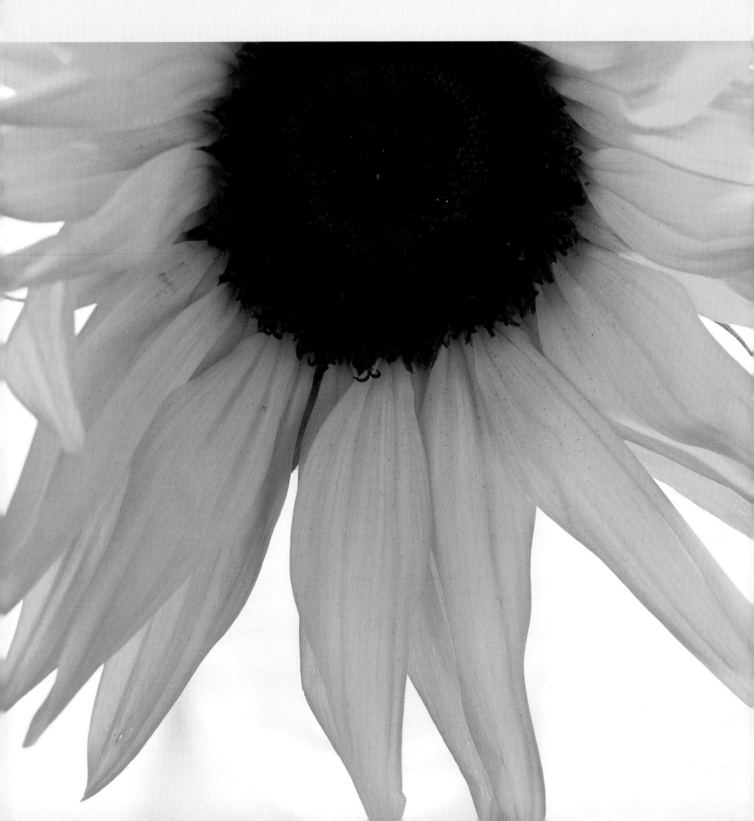

REFRESH & REVIVE

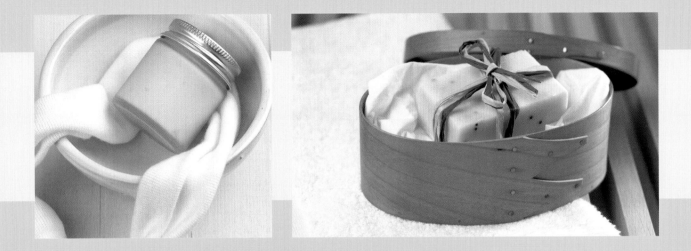

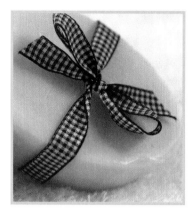

SUNNY SOAP

Ingredients

11 fl oz mineral water

A handful each of lavatera and chamomile flowers

8 fl oz sunflower oil

8 fl oz pomace or olive oil

7 oz coconut oil

4 oz caustic soda

2 tsp bergamot essential oil

1 tsp sweet orange essential oil

1 tsp ylang ylang essential oil

$^1/_2$ tsp tangerine essential oil

Equipment

General equipment (see page 12)

Safety equipment (see page 13)

Sieve

Wooden board

Tray

Method

1 Work in a well-ventilated room. Oil and line a plastic mold with waxed paper.

2 Prepare the mineral water by boiling and infusing the chamomile and lavatera flowers (see page 20). Allow to cool completely, then strain and reserve the infusion and the flowers.

3 Melt the sunflower, pomace, and coconut oils in a large stainless-steel saucepan over low heat.

4 Wearing protective goggles, a mask, an apron, and long rubber gloves, add the caustic soda to the infused mineral water in a tall plastic bucket. Stir with a plastic spatula until dissolved.

5 Using one jam thermometer for the oils and another for the caustic soda mixture (lye water), monitor both solutions until they reach 96°F. Still wearing the protective clothing, immediately pour the lye water into the oils. Continuously stir for approximately 15 minutes with the spatula; you will see the mixture thickening.

6 Tracing occurs when a drizzle of the mixture on the surface of the soap leaves a visible line. At this point, pour in the essential oils and combine thoroughly. Add half of the chamomile and lavatera flowers to give texture and mix until evenly distributed.

7 Pour the soap mixture into the prepared mold and place in a safe, warm, dry place for 24 hours, covering with cardboard to keep the heat in.

8 Wearing protective gloves—the soap is still caustic at this point—turn the soap out onto a wooden board covered with waxed paper. Peel off the lining paper and cut the bar into the desired shapes using a carving knife or cookie cutters. If the mixture is too soft to cut, leave for another 24 hours. Space out the cut soaps on waxed paper in a tray and leave in a dark, warm, dry place for four weeks to mature, turning several times.

This easy-to-make soap has a base of **sunflower** oil and pomace oil. Pomace oil is the last pressing of olive oil and speeds up the tracing time of the soap. However, if you can't find it in the supermarket, you can use normal olive oil instead. **Coconut oil** is added for lather and its moisturizing properties. A blend of citrus essential oils contains bergamot, which is **stimulating** to those early morning senses, and sweet orange oil, for a real sunshine feeling and aroma. Sensual **ylang ylang** will leave you feeling fresh and in a good mood all day.

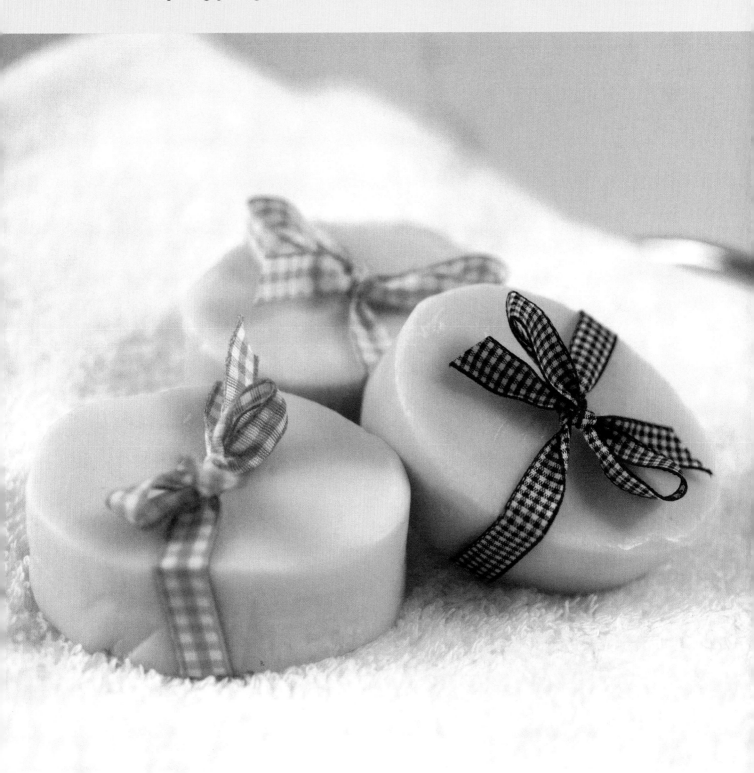

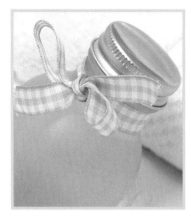

The **zingy**, zesty combination of grapefruit and mandarin essential oils will really **wake you up** in the morning and leave a wonderful fresh aroma on the skin.

Lavender and mandarin are excellent **essential oils** for **sensitive** skins. This delicious oil also has useful insect-repellent properties for the hot summer months.

WIDE-AWAKE MASSAGE OIL

Ingredients

9 fl oz sweet almond oil

5 drops grapefruit essential oil

10 drops mandarin essential oil

2 drops lavender essential oil

Equipment

Dark or clear glass bottle with tight-fitting lid

Method

1 Pour all the ingredients into a dark or clear glass bottle and shake gently to mix. A clear glass bottle should be stored in a dark place to protect the essential oils from light.

2 Rub the oil into the skin in the morning and imagine you are waking up to the scent of lavender fields wafting on a gentle Mediterranean breeze, looking out over orchards of almonds and oranges.

Safety consideration

If you have a serious nut allergy, you will need to replace the sweet almond oil. Grapeseed and sunflower oils make good alternatives.

Do not use citrus essential oils if you are likely to be exposed to the sun, since it makes the skin more sensitive to sunlight.

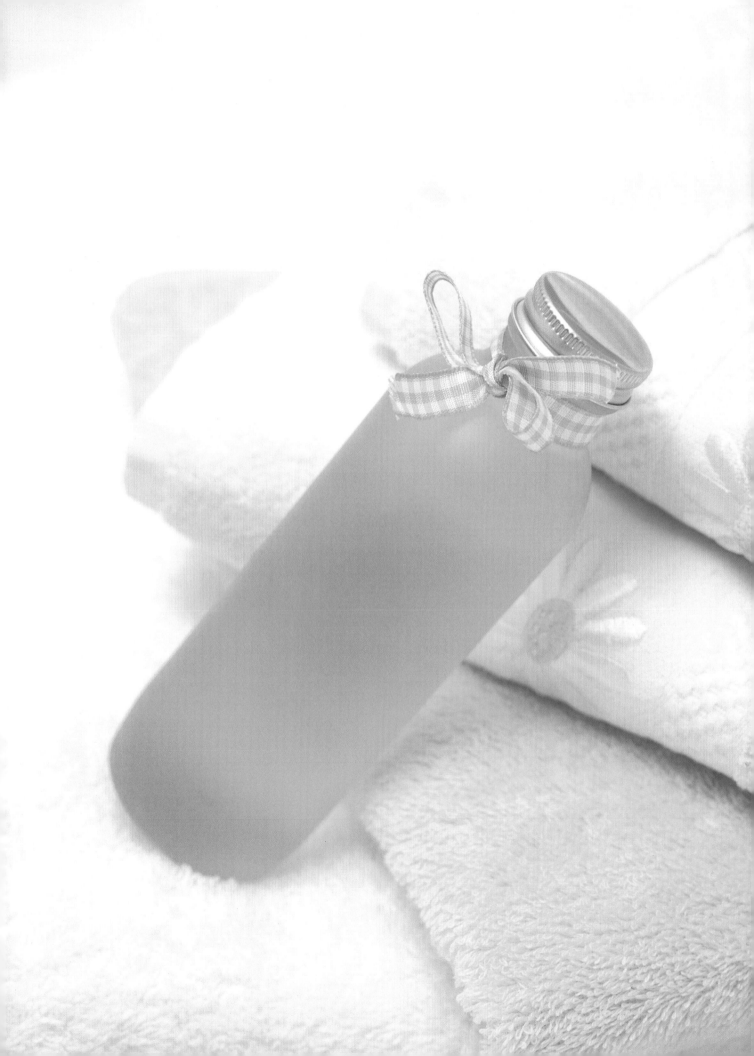

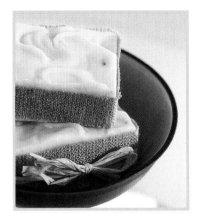

MORNING GLORY SOAP

Ingredients

7 fl oz pomace or olive oil

4 fl oz sweet almond oil

3 fl oz sunflower oil

2$\frac{1}{2}$ oz coconut oil

2$\frac{1}{2}$ oz palm oil

1 fl oz calendula oil

1$\frac{1}{2}$ oz beeswax

2$\frac{1}{2}$ oz caustic soda

8 fl oz mineral water

1 tsp lime essential oil

1 tsp sweet orange essential oil

1 tsp may chang essential oil

$\frac{1}{2}$ tsp frankincense essential oil

Petals from 20 dried calendula flowers

Equipment

General equipment (see page 12)

Safety equipment (see page 13)

Wooden board

Tray

Method

1 Work in a well-ventilated room. Oil and line a plastic mold with waxed paper.

2 Melt the pomace, sweet almond, sunflower, coconut, palm, and calendula oils with the beeswax in a large stainless-steel saucepan over low heat.

3 Wearing protective goggles, a mask, an apron, and long rubber gloves, pour the caustic soda into the mineral water in a tall plastic bucket, and stir with a plastic spatula to dissolve.

4 Using one jam thermometer for the oils and one for the caustic soda mixture (lye water), monitor each mix until they both reach 131°F.

5 Still wearing the protective clothing, immediately pour the lye water into the oils. Continuously stir with the spatula for approximately 15 minutes; you will see the mixture thickening.

6 Tracing occurs when a drizzle of the mixture on the surface of the soap leaves a visible line. At this point, pour in the essential oils and mix well. Add the calendula petals and stir until evenly distributed.

7 Pour the soap into the prepared mold. At this stage, the soap is thick enough to have a pattern made across its surface. Drag a fork across the top to make a ripple pattern, first one way and then the other, or design your own motif.

8 Leave to set in a warm, dry place, covered with cardboard to keep the heat in. After 24 hours, turn it out onto a wooden board covered with waxed paper. The soap is still caustic at this stage, so wear gloves to peel off the soap's lining paper, then use a carving knife to cut it into chunky bars of approximately 4 oz, or $\frac{1}{4}$ lb, each. Set out the soaps on a tray lined with waxed paper and leave to mature for four weeks in a dry, warm place, turning occasionally.

Use this soap first thing and you'll be ready to take on the world! It is a **deliciously indulgent** blend of skin-conditioning essential oils. What's more, there's no need to moisturize after using this one. Calendula oil and **sweet orange** essential oil are known for their healing properties and will leave your skin feeling silky soft throughout the day. Frankincense has been used for centuries as an antiseptic with powers to neutralize offensive odors, while lime and may chang are **reviving** oils and will add an exotic touch to your morning shower.

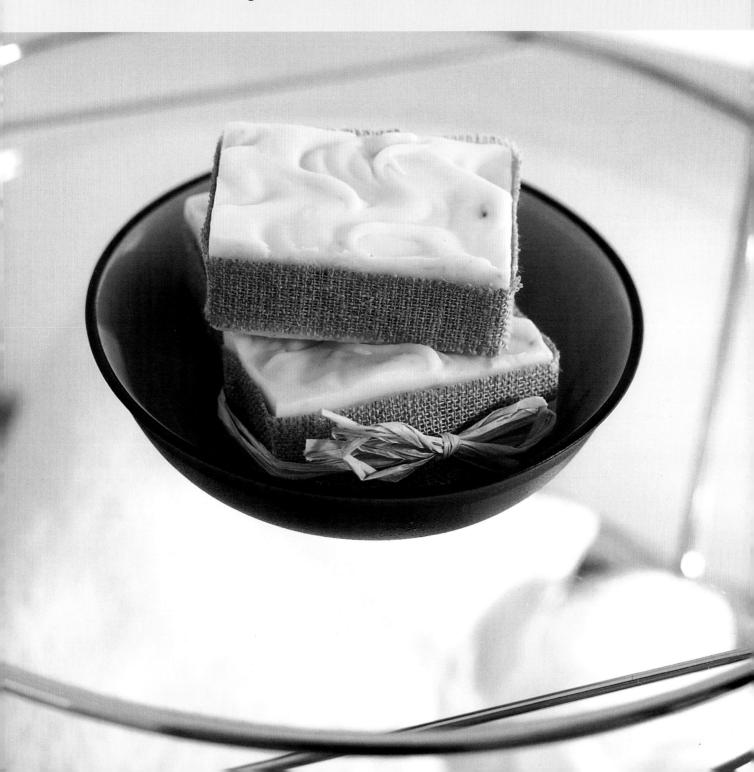

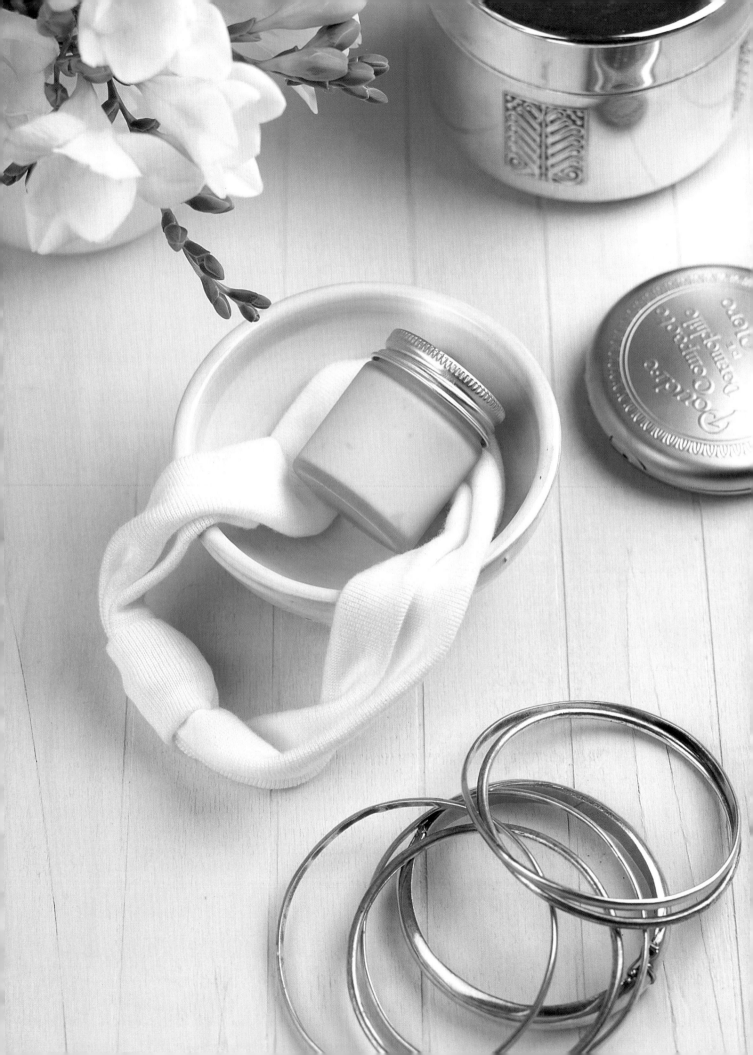

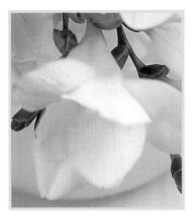

Most skins will benefit from this healthy mixture of avocado oil and **sweet almond oil.** We have added lemon and geranium essential oils, not just for their benefits in **revitalizing** and **refreshing** the skin but for their wonderfully uplifting aroma.

If you are a sun worshiper, replace the lemon oil with lavender (see note about **citrus oils** on page 17).

MEGA MOISTURIZING CREAM

Ingredients

1½ fl oz sweet almond oil

1 fl oz avocado oil

½ oz beeswax

2 Tbsp mineral water

2 drops lemon essential oil

1 drop geranium essential oil

Equipment

Stainless-steel saucepan

Wooden spoon

Dark or clear glass jar with lids

Method

1 Melt the oils and beeswax together in a heavy-bottomed stainless-steel pan. Warm the water and beat it slowly into the mixture.

2 Remove from the heat and stir until the cream cools to body temperature. Stir in the essential oils and combine thoroughly to make a smooth cream.

3 Spoon into glass jars and shake until the lotion has cooled completely, to stop the oil and water from separating. Store clear glass jars in a dark place to protect the essential oils from light.

KEEN AS MUSTARD SOAP

Ingredients

7 fl oz extra-virgin olive oil

4 fl oz sunflower oil

2$\frac{1}{2}$ oz palm oil

2$\frac{1}{2}$ oz coconut oil

1 fl oz sweet almond oil

1$\frac{1}{2}$ oz beeswax

2$\frac{1}{2}$ oz caustic soda

8 fl oz mineral water

2 tsp lemongrass essential oil

1 tsp lime essential oil

$\frac{1}{2}$ tsp rosemary essential oil

2 drops benzoin essential oil

2 Tbsp mustard seeds

Equipment

General equipment (see page 12)

Safety equipment (see page 13)

Wooden board

Tray

Method

1. Work in a well-ventilated area. Oil and line a plastic mold with waxed paper.

2. Melt the olive, sunflower, palm, coconut, and sweet almond oils with the beeswax in a large stainless-steel saucepan over low heat.

3. Wearing protective goggles, a mask, an apron, and long rubber gloves, pour the caustic soda into the mineral water in a tall plastic bucket. Stir with a plastic spatula until dissolved.

4. Using one jam thermometer for the oils and another for the caustic soda mixture (lye water), let both solutions reach 131°F. At this point, wearing the protective clothing, pour the lye water into the oils and combine thoroughly with the spatula.

5. Keep stirring until tracing occurs—when a drizzle of the mixture on the surface of the soap leaves a visible line. Add the essential oils and then the mustard seeds, mixing well.

6. Pour into the prepared mold and leave for 24 hours, covered with cardboard, in a dry, warm place.

7. Wearing rubber gloves, turn out the soap onto a wooden board covered with waxed paper. Cut into bars with a carving knife and space out on a tray lined with waxed paper in a warm, dark place for four weeks, turning regularly.

8. Use before a busy day or a night out, to give you extra energy.

A vacation favorite
Lemongrass and lime essential oils are both natural insect repellants, so this is great to use during the summer or to take on warm-weather vacations.

Fabulous in the shower and with an aroma loved equally by men and women, this soap is a sizzling mixture of lime and lemongrass essential oils (to **freshen** the body) and rosemary (to revive the senses). Lemongrass has a stimulating effect on the whole system and has antiseptic and deodorizing properties, and **rosemary** is a real wake-up oil. Used for many centuries in medicines, rosemary will revive your senses, both physical and mental. The joy of this soap is the real mustard seeds, which will smooth your rough edges with a **gentle** exfoliating action.

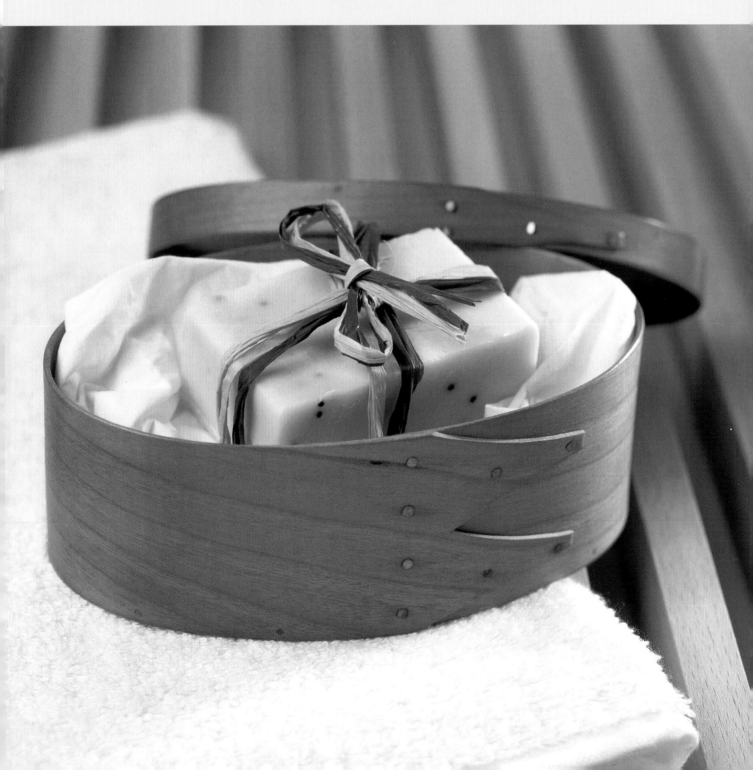

For many men, the days of a leisurely shave with brush and bowl are gone. Instead, shaving is part of their shower routine. So we have come up with this delectably moisturizing soap that combines the emollient properties of avocado oil with the freshness of cedarwood and clary sage essential oils, revered for their nutty aromas and skin-conditioning properties. Both oils have aphrodisiac properties and will give off a sexy, masculine feeling to start the day.

SMOOTHING SHAVE SOAP

Ingredients

9 fl oz olive oil

3 fl oz avocado oil

2$\frac{1}{2}$ oz coconut oil

1$\frac{1}{2}$ oz palm oil

1$\frac{1}{2}$ oz beeswax

1 oz cocoa butter

2$\frac{1}{2}$ oz caustic soda

8 fl oz mineral water

3 tsp clary sage essential oil

1 tsp cedarwood essential oil

Equipment

General equipment (see page 12)

Safety equipment (see page 13)

Wooden board

Tray

Method

1 Work in a well-ventilated room. Oil a plastic mold and line with waxed paper.

2 Melt the olive, avocado, coconut, and palm oils with the beeswax and cocoa butter in a large stainless-steel saucepan over low heat.

3 Wearing protective eyewear, a mask, an apron, and long rubber gloves, pour the mineral water into a tall plastic bucket and slowly pour in the caustic soda, stirring to dissolve using a plastic spatula.

4 Use one jam thermometer for the caustic soda mix (lye water) and one for the oil mixture. Monitor both mixtures until they equalize at 131°F. Wearing the protective clothing, immediately pour the lye water into the oils, stirring continuously with the spatula until well combined.

5 Continue stirring until tracing occurs (see page 11), then pour in the essential oils and stir in thoroughly. Pour the mixture into the prepared mold. Swirl the surface with the spatula if you are going to cut the soap into bars, or leave it smooth.

6 Leave to set in a warm, dry place for 24 hours, covered with cardboard to keep the heat in. Wearing protective gloves, turn the soap out onto a wooden board lined with waxed paper and cut into bars or rounds with a carving knife or cookie cutter. Set out the soaps on a tray lined with waxed paper and leave in a warm, dry place for four weeks to mature, turning occasionally.

> **One for the shaving bowl**
> If you use a shaving bowl, simply make up the soap as normal, then, when it is set, use a round cutter that is just smaller in diameter than the bowl.

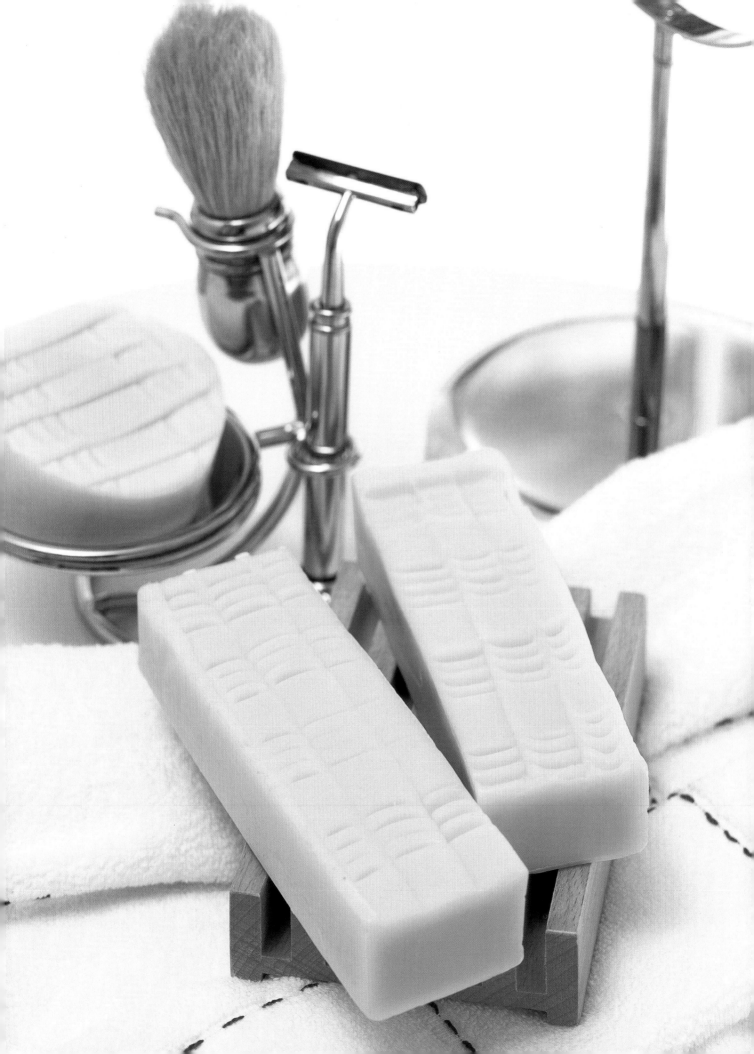

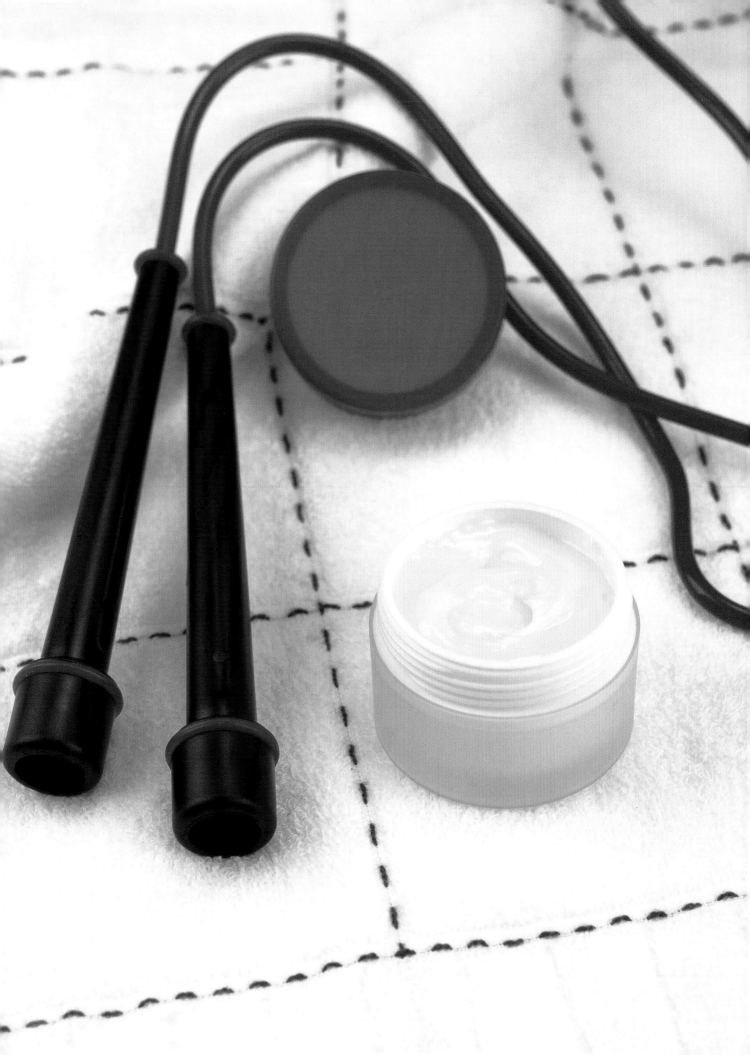

Black pepper, as you would expect, has a **powerful** stimulant effect, a property that is put to very good use in this presport rub. Combined with **rosemary**, the wake-up herb, these essential oils will also sharpen your concentration and help your joints and muscles cope with the demands of exercise, minimizing pain and stiffness afterward. As this is designed to improve **performance** and prevent fatigue, no sportsman or sportswoman can afford to leave home without this magical cream.

SPRINT PRE-EXERCISE MASSAGE CREAM

Ingredients

2 oz coconut oil

1 fl oz sweet almond oil

$1/2$ oz beeswax

$1/2$ oz cocoa butter

$2^1/2$ fl oz mineral water

$1^1/2$ tsp rosemary essential oil

$1/2$ tsp black pepper essential oil

Equipment

Stainless-steel saucepan

Wooden spoon

Dark or clear glass jars with lids

Method

1. Place the coconut and sweet almond oils in a heavy-bottomed stainless-steel saucepan with the beeswax and cocoa butter. Gently melt them over low heat. Beat in the mineral water with a wooden spoon until a smooth cream is obtained.

2. Remove from the heat and keep stirring until the cream has cooled to body temperature. Stir in the essential oils.

3. Spoon into glass jars and shake until the lotion has cooled completely, to stop the oil and water from separating. Store clear jars in a dark place to preserve the oils.

4. Your mind and body will be ready for any kind of action after rubbing this one on!

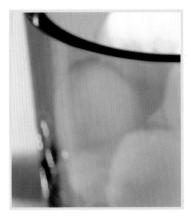

Ahh, **peppermint**! If ever there were an essential oil to put a spring in your step, this is it. Peppermint—with its **cooling**, refreshing, and **energizing** properties—will stimulate your mind and body, wake you up, and prepare your feet for the rigors of the day.

Thyme essential oil has been added as an antiseptic and because it **fights fatigue**. This cream is definitely not one to use at bedtime.

COOL-AND-MINTY FOOT CREAM

Ingredients

2 oz coconut oil

1 fl oz calendula oil

1/2 oz beeswax

1/2 oz cocoa butter

2 1/2 fl oz mineral water

1 1/2 tsp peppermint essential oil

1/2 tsp thyme essential oil

Equipment

Stainless-steel saucepan

Wooden spoon

Dark or clear glass jars with lids

Method

1 Place the coconut and calendula oils in a heavy-bottomed stainless-steel saucepan with the beeswax and cocoa butter. Gently melt them over low heat. Beat in the mineral water with a wooden spoon.

2 Remove from the heat and stir until the cream cools to body temperature. Stir in the essential oils, making sure that they are thoroughly combined to make a smooth cream.

3 Spoon into glass jars and shake until the lotion has cooled completely, to stop the oil and water from separating. Store clear glass jars in a dark place to protect the essential oils from light.

4 Rub into the feet first thing in the morning or in preparation for a night out dancing. If you love the aroma as much as we do, you can actually use it all over and it will leave the skin feeling cool and refreshed.

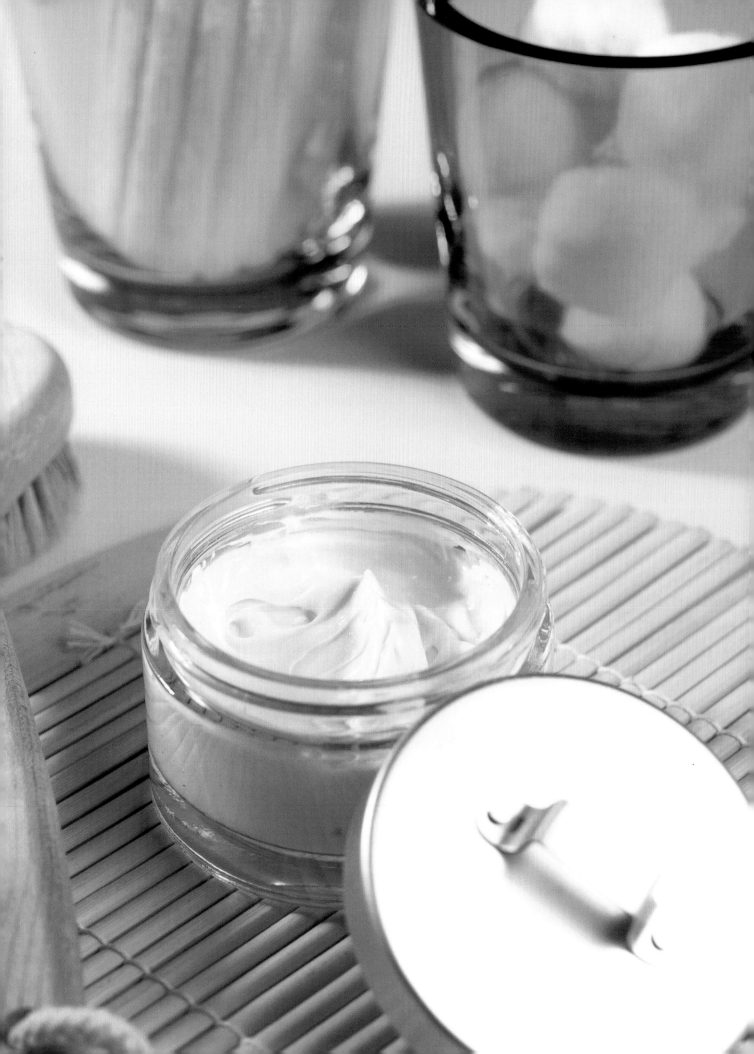

HAIR BARE SHAMPOO BAR

Ingredients

1 pint olive oil

3$\frac{1}{2}$ fl oz sweet almond oil

2$\frac{1}{2}$ oz beeswax

2 oz coconut cream oil

9 fl oz mineral water

Six handfuls of nettle tops

4$\frac{1}{2}$ oz caustic soda

1 fl oz bergamot essential oil

1$\frac{1}{2}$ tsp lavender essential oil

1$\frac{1}{2}$ tsp lemongrass essential oil

Equipment

General equipment (see page 12)

Safety equipment (see page 13)

Sieve

Wooden board

Tray

Method

1 Work in a well-ventilated room. Oil and line a plastic mold with waxed paper.

2 Prepare the mineral water by boiling and infusing the nettle tops (see page 20). Allow to cool completely, then strain and reserve the infusion. Chop the infused nettles finely and set aside.

3 Melt the olive and sweet almond oils with the beeswax and coconut cream oil in a large stainless-steel saucepan over low heat. Stir well using a stainless-steel spoon, and do not allow the coconut cream oil to "catch" on the bottom.

4 Wearing protective goggles, a mask, an apron, and long rubber gloves, add the caustic soda to the infused mineral water in a tall plastic bucket. Stir with a plastic spatula until dissolved.

5 Using one jam thermometer for the oils and another for the caustic soda mixture (lye water), allow both solutions to reach 131°F. At this point, still wearing the protective clothing, pour the lye water into the oil mixture, stirring continuously with the spatula.

6 Keep stirring until the solution traces—when a drizzle of mixture leaves a line on the surface of the soap. Pour in the essential oils, thoroughly incorporating them into the soap. Add the chopped nettles and stir.

7 Pour the soap into the prepared mold, cover with cardboard, and leave in a safe, warm, dry place for 24 hours.

8 Wearing protective gloves, turn the soap out onto a wooden board covered with waxed paper. Peel off the lining paper and cut the soap into the desired shapes using a carving knife or cookie cutters. Space the cut soaps out on a tray lined with waxed paper and leave to mature for four weeks in a dry, dark place, turning several times.

Hair rinsed in an infusion of nettles will be shiny and well conditioned, a property we capitalize on with this shampoo bar. The basis of this soap is an infusion of young nettle tips in mineral water. This is combined with bergamot, lavender, and lemongrass essential oils to stimulate the scalp, prevent dandruff and flakiness, and impart a delightful citrus aroma.

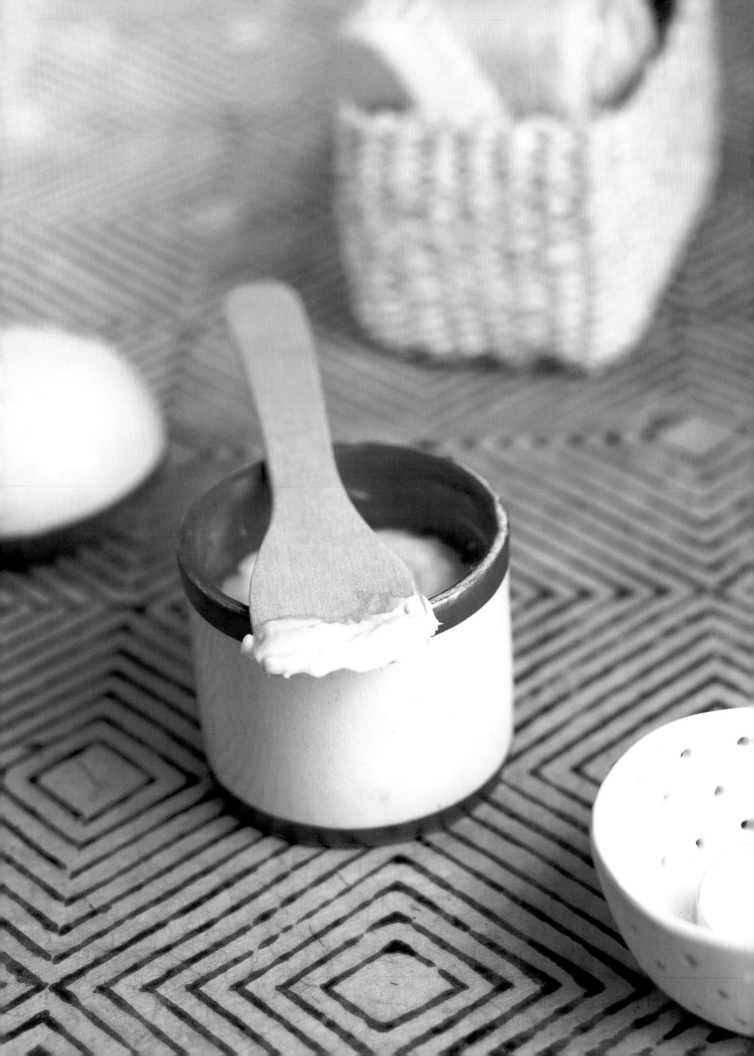

More and more men are overcoming their fears when it comes to using **moisturizers**. The combination of bay, cedarwood, and clary sage essential oils in this moisturizer, designed specifically for men, is a classic and leaves a lingering but not too overpowering aroma. Bay has great **healing** and antiseptic properties—to soothe skin irritated after shaving—and a spicy, masculine fragrance, ideal for men's toiletries. An herbal infusion is included and can be varied according to skin type. Chamomile is useful for irritated, inflamed skin; calendula flowers for combination skin; elderflowers for sallow skin; and lemon balm leaves or lime flowers for **all skin types**.

BAYWATCH FACE CREAM FOR MEN

Ingredients

A handful of dried flowers, such as chamomile, calendula, or elderflower

³/₄ oz beeswax

1 fl oz rosehip oil

1¹/₂ fl oz sweet almond oil

10 drops clary sage essential oil

4 drops cedarwood essential oil

2 drops bay essential oil

Equipment

Measuring jug

Sieve

Stainless-steel saucepan

Wooden spoon

Dark or clear glass jars with lids

Method

1 Make an herbal infusion with the dried flowers and 10 fl oz boiling water (see page 20). Strain and set aside to cool.

2 Melt the beeswax in a heavy-bottomed stainless-steel saucepan, then add the rosehip and sweet almond oils, beating steadily with a wooden spoon. Add 1¹/₂ fl oz of the herbal infusion in a slow trickle.

3 Take the saucepan off the heat and continue to stir until the lotion has cooled to body temperature. Stir in the essential oils.

4 Decant the cream into glass jars and place the lids on tightly. Now shake the mixture until the lotion has entirely cooled—this process will prevent the oil and water from separating. Store clear glass jars in a dark place to preserve the essential oils.

5 Use in the morning or before bed to give your face some love and attention.

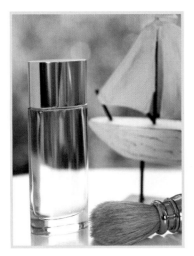

There are many and varied brands of aftershave on the market, but if you want to really **look after your skin**, it is nice to know exactly what goes into the product, or—even better—to make your own. The essential oils in this aftershave splash have been chosen for their **therapeutic** values and lasting, but not overpowering, aromas. You can use them as suggested or **mix** them to your own preference, within the suggested quantities.

CLOSE-SHAVE AFTERSHAVE SPLASH

Ingredients

1 fl oz vodka

9 fl oz witch hazel

3 drops bay essential oil

*3 drops lime essential oil
or 1 fl oz vodka*

3 drops bergamot essential oil

3 drops cedarwood essential oil

Equipment

*Dark or clear glass bottle with
tight-fitting lid*

Method

1 Mix together all the ingredients in a dark or clear glass bottle with a lid. If using a clear glass bottle, remember to store the mix in a dark place to ensure the essential oils are well preserved.

2 Shake the mixture well before use, then simply pour a little into the hand and splash away.

Therapeutic benefits

Bay essential oil is antiseptic and bactericidal, while lime has a cooling, refreshing aroma and uplifts the spirits. The essential oil of bergamot is a mood-enhancer guaranteed to leave you with a spring in your step and a smile on your face. Cedarwood's use in skin preparations for men reflects its antiseptic and astringent properties and its masculine aroma (with a reputation as an aphrodisiac, too).

Witch hazel is a tonic and astringent as well as a sedative—and so wonderfully soothing. Vodka gives the great cool, tingly feeling that every good aftershave should give, and the cheapest brand will do.

Safety consideration

Citrus essential oils make the skin more sensitive to sunlight, so do not use them if you are likely to be exposed to the sun.

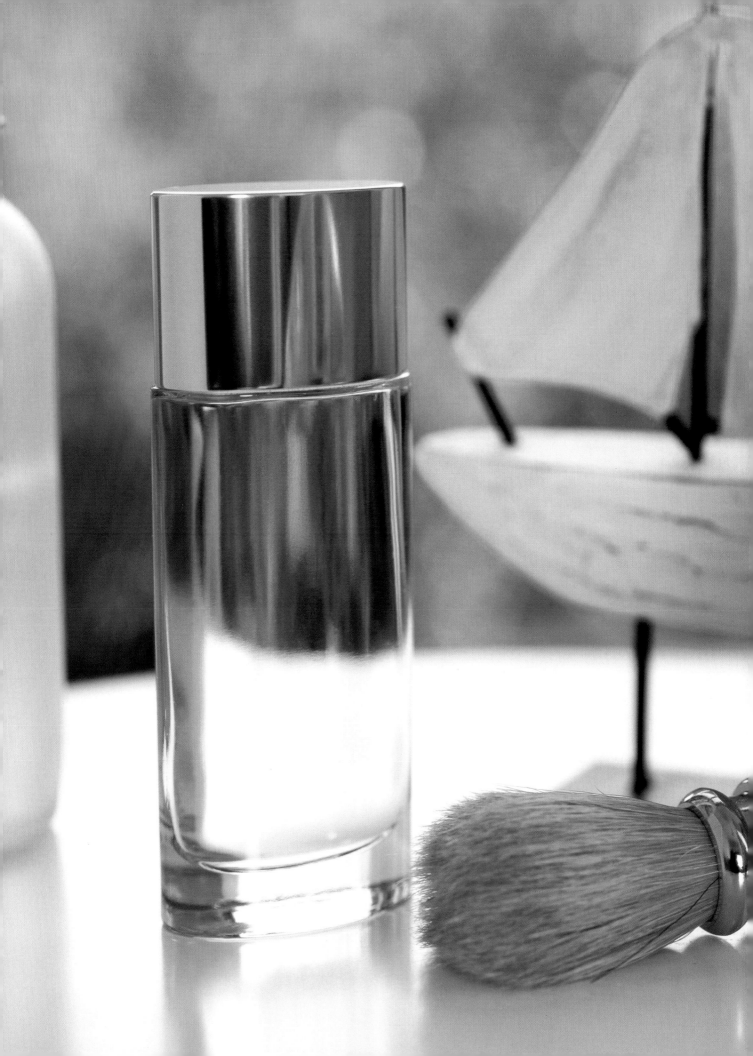

GIFTWRAPPING IDEAS

These soaps and other bathroom gifts look wonderful when wrapped in brightly colored ribbons.

Why not package up one of the soaps with a soft facecloth to make a really special gift? Tissue

paper, cellophane, and sheer fabric are all pretty ways of wrapping items. Corrugated cardboard

not only protects glass bottles but makes an alternative wrapping, especially when decorated with

a slice of dried fruit.

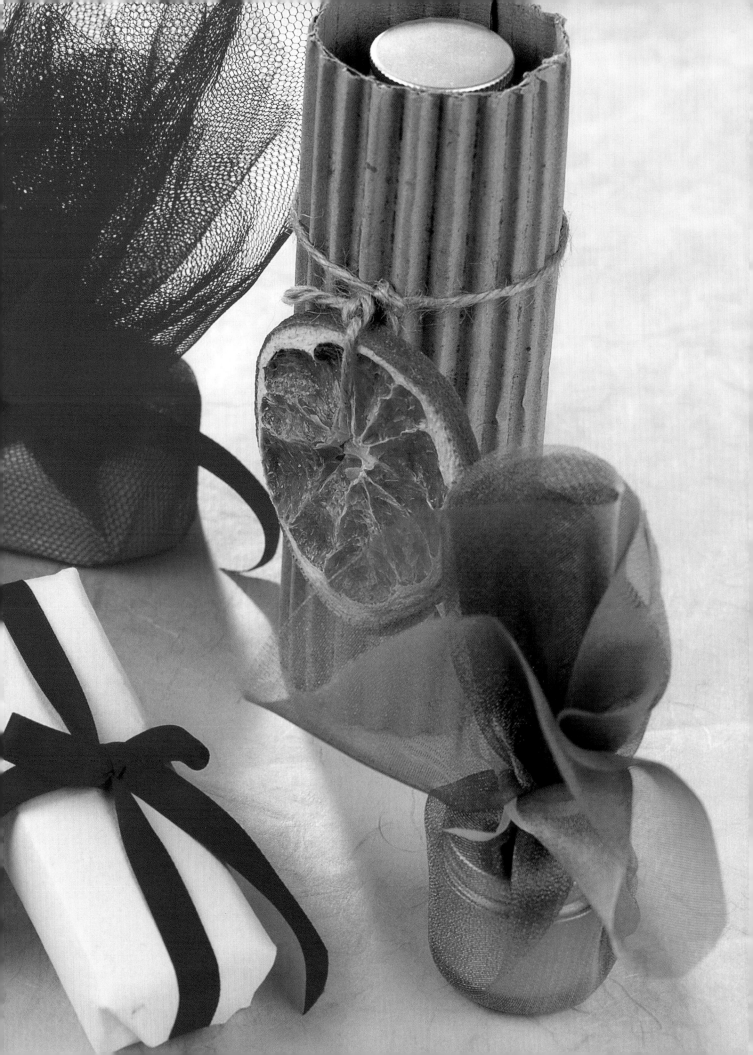

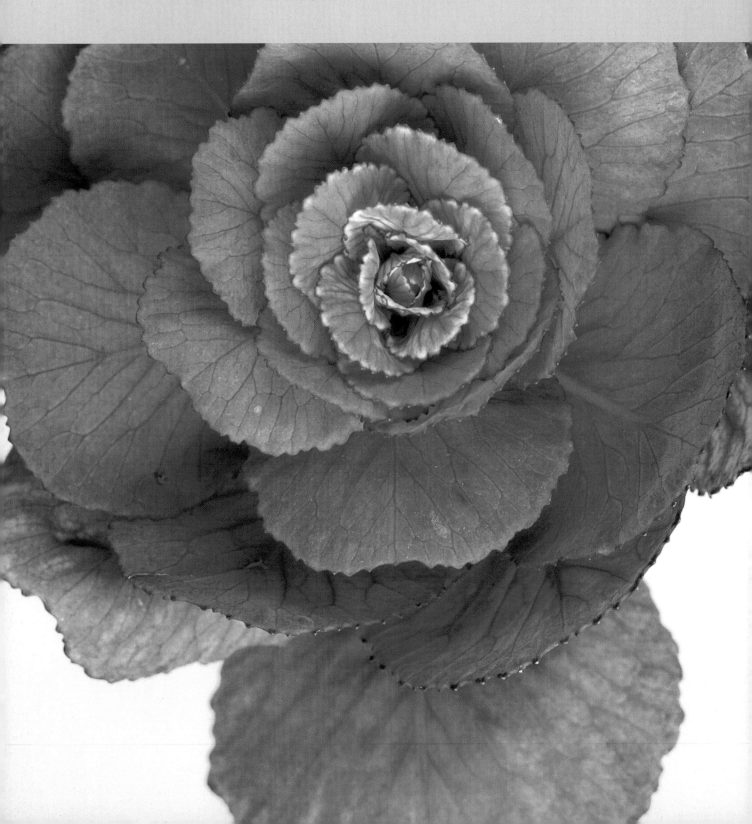

PAMPER & INDULGE

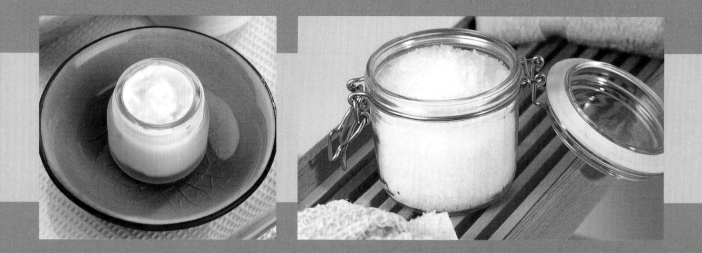

Summertime is exposure time for feet, which could be embarrassing if yours have hard skin, cracked heels, or discolored nails. In this case, drastic measures are needed, so we have pulled out all the stops. Tried and tested on the most horrible of tootsies, this foot scrub will transform not only their look but also their smell.

WELL-HEELED FOOT SCRUB

Ingredients

4 fl oz sweet almond oil

8 drops lemon essential oil

4 drops tea tree essential oil

2 drops myrrh essential oil

7 oz Maldon salt flakes

Equipment

Mixing bowl

Spoon

Dark or clear glass jars with lids

Method

1 Mix together the sweet almond oil and essential oils, then add the salt and stir well. Keep in dark jars or store the scrub in clear glass jars in a dark place, to ensure that the aroma is preserved.

2 Before using the scrub, wash your feet and soak them in warm water for about five minutes, to soften the skin. Dry the feet, then scoop out a handful of scrub and, keeping the foot over a bowl or bath to avoid making a mess, massage all over the foot, paying particular attention to areas of hard skin. Rinse the salt off with tepid water, then pat dry with a soft towel. Your feet will never have felt so good. Put on a pair of cotton socks that will allow the oils to sink in and do their job without leaving greasy, slippery footprints.

A treat for feet

Lemon essential oil is enormously beneficial for feet. Having a mild bleaching action to revive skin, it aids brittle nails, treats corns, stimulates the circulation, and helps to rid the body of acidity—in cases of gout, for instance. Tea tree is a powerful antiseptic and, when blended with lemon essential oil, yields an aroma that is a truly magical combination. A couple of drops of myrrh essential oil make a useful addition to this scrub because myrrh is antifungal, particularly useful to feet in hot weather.

Safety consideration

Do not use myrrh essential oil while pregnant. If you're expecting, simply remove the myrrh from this recipe.

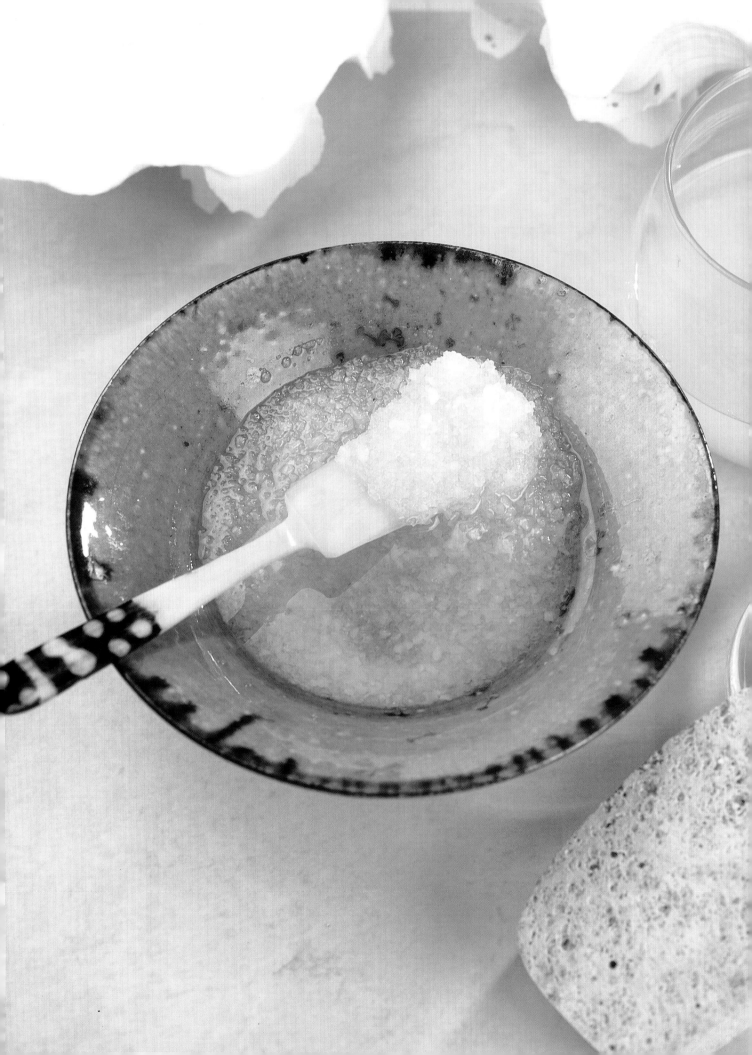

BAYSIC INSTINCT SOAP FOR MEN

Ingredients

A handful of bay leaves

8 fl oz sunflower oil

8 fl oz olive oil

7 oz coconut oil

4 oz caustic soda

11 fl oz mineral water

2 tsp bergamot essential oil

1 1/2 tsp bay essential oil

1 tsp patchouli essential oil

1/2 tsp cinnamon essential oil

Equipment

General equipment (see page 12)

Safety equipment (see page 13)

Wooden board

Tray

Method

1 Work in a well-ventilated area. Oil and line a plastic mold with waxed paper.

2 If you don't have a bay tree in the garden, bay leaves are readily available fresh or dried at the supermarket. Chop a handful of leaves very small, removing and discarding the veins.

3 Melt the sunflower, olive, and coconut oils together in a large stainless-steel saucepan over low heat.

4 Wearing protective goggles, a face mask, an apron, and long rubber gloves, add the caustic soda to the mineral water in a tall plastic bucket and stir well with a plastic spatula until thoroughly dissolved.

5 Using one jam thermometer for the oils and another for the caustic soda mixture (lye water), allow both solutions to reach 96°F. Still wearing the protective clothing, immediately pour the lye water into the oils and stir thoroughly. Continue stirring with the spatula until the mixture traces—when a drizzle of the mix leaves a visible line on the surface of the soap.

6 Now add the essential oils and chopped bay leaves, mixing them evenly into the soap.

7 Pour the soap into the prepared mold, cover with cardboard to keep the heat in, and leave in a warm, dry, safe place for 24 hours.

8 Wearing protective gloves, turn out the soap onto a wooden board covered with waxed paper. Peel off the lining paper and cut into chunky bars using a carving knife. Lay the soaps on a tray covered with waxed paper, spacing them to allow for air circulation. Store in a dark, dry, warm place for four weeks, turning several times during the maturing process.

This soap is dedicated to Eva French, a **wonderful** Jamaican lady from New York, who so impressed Ada with her relaxed Caribbean style that we created this soap in her honor. The rich, **warm aroma** of bay leaves is the essence of Bay Rum, the traditional cologne of the West Indies. In Ancient Greece, sporting champions were crowned with bay leaves—what better scent, then, could there be to give a heroic husband or boyfriend. Combining fresh bay leaves with bay, bergamot, cinnamon, and **patchouli** essential oils makes a fresh ultramasculine soap.

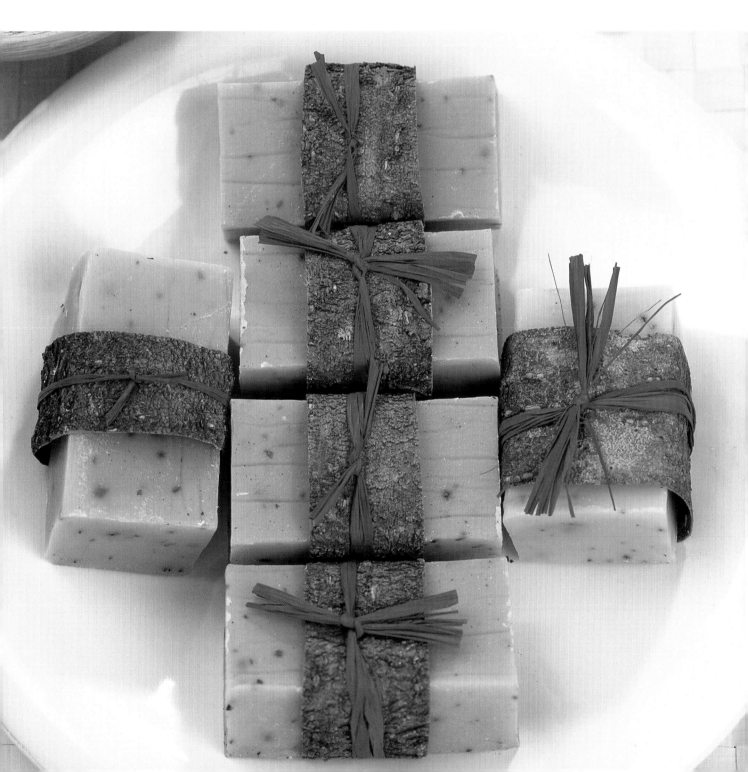

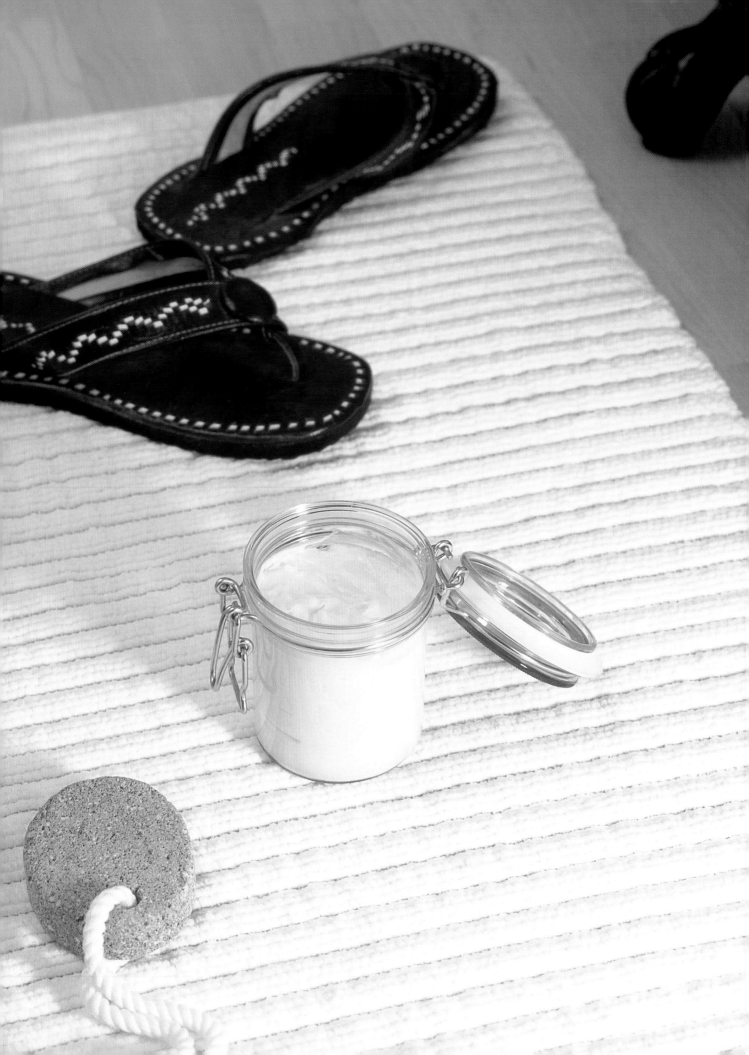

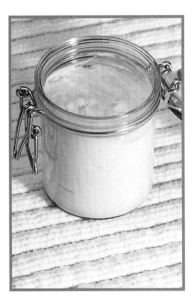

Feet are not the most glamorous part of the body, but we would be lost without them, so it pays to heed the following advice: take the time to **relax** your feet (see below), then massage them with this delicious combination of lemongrass, sage, and rosemary essential oils in an ultra-moisturizing base. Sage will deal with any problems of sweatiness, while rosemary **revives**—and, as a bonus, they are both great for relieving aches and pains. Lemongrass has an amazingly fresh aroma and will **stimulate** the circulation as well as being a **powerful** antiseptic and

FOOTLOOSE FOOT LOTION

Ingredients

¹/₂ oz beeswax

¹/₂ oz cocoa butter

2 oz coconut oil

2 Tbsp sweet almond oil

2 fl oz mineral water

1 tsp lemongrass essential oil

¹/₂ tsp sage essential oil

¹/₂ tsp rosemary essential oil

Equipment

Stainless-steel saucepan

Wooden spoon

Dark or clear glass jar with lid

Method

1 Place the beeswax, cocoa butter, and the coconut and sweet almond oils in a heavy-bottomed stainless-steel saucepan and melt slowly over low heat. Thoroughly beat in the mineral water with a wooden spoon until a smooth mixture is obtained.

2 Take the boiler off the heat and keep stirring until the cream has cooled to body temperature. Add the essential oils and mix thoroughly.

3 Decant the cream to airtight jars and shake until the lotion has cooled completely, to stop the oil and water from separating. Store clear glass jars in a dark place.

Massaging the feet
At the end of a tiring day, the best thing you can do is put your feet up, preferably by lying down with your feet higher than your heart, making sure that the whole leg is well supported. This greatly assists the circulation—including that of the lymphatic system—and relieves swelling and the feeling of heaviness in the legs. Very gentle massage toward the heart, using either the fingertips or a relaxed hand, will increase the beneficial effect of raising the legs.

It is reputed that West African women tie ginger to their husbands' belts to revive their men's sexual prowess. Which is where the "What Women Want" bit comes from! We can't guarantee the effectiveness in this case, but the ginger in these bath salts will certainly revive any man who comes home from work and collapses in a chair in front of the television.

Lemongrass essential oil gives an instant lift and will wash any sticky sweatiness away. It also soothes headaches and stimulates the whole body, just the thing after a hard day at work. These salts are very quick to make, and it is better to prep a small quantity at a time so that they are always fresh.

"WHAT WOMEN WANT" BATH SALTS FOR MEN

Ingredients
1 tsp sweet almond oil
6 drops lemongrass essential oil
3 drops ginger essential oil
4 oz Dead Sea salt

Equipment
Mixing bowl
Spoon
Dark or clear glass jars with lids

Method

1 Mix together the sweet almond oil and the essential oils, then stir in the Dead Sea salt. Pour into dark glass jars with lids or keep clear glass jars in a dark place to protect the mix from light.

2 Take a warm, refreshing bath with these energizing salts and see how much better you feel—one heaped teaspoonful added to your bath should do the trick. The salts are best used within a couple of months, but they are so good that we're sure they will be used up well before then.

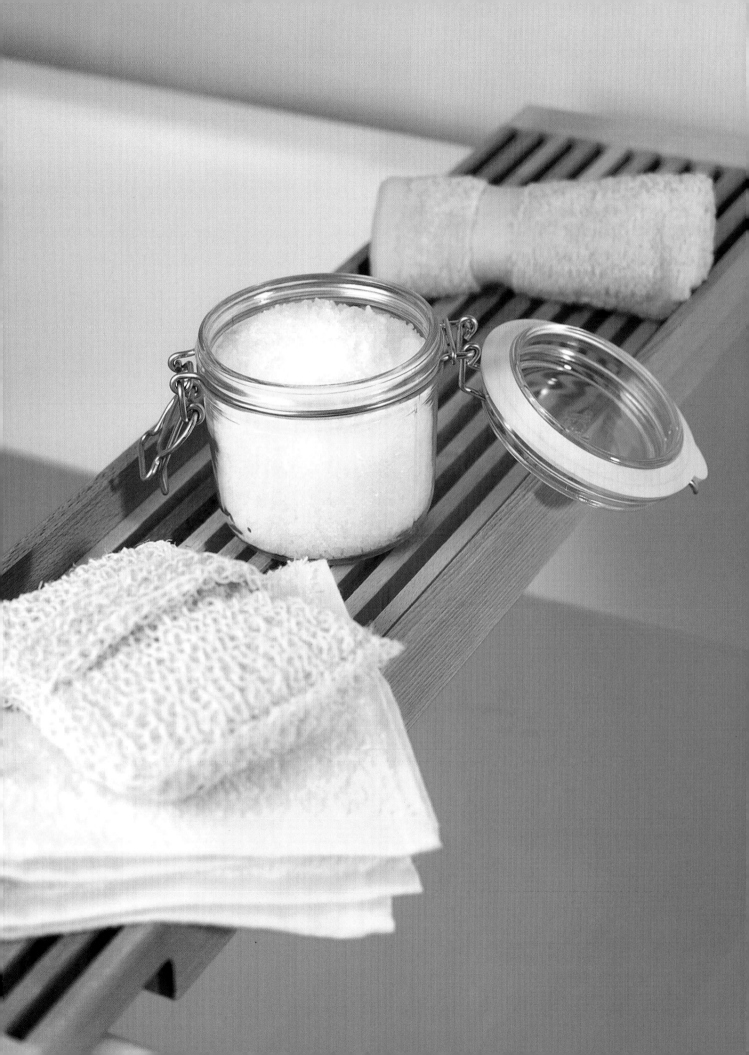

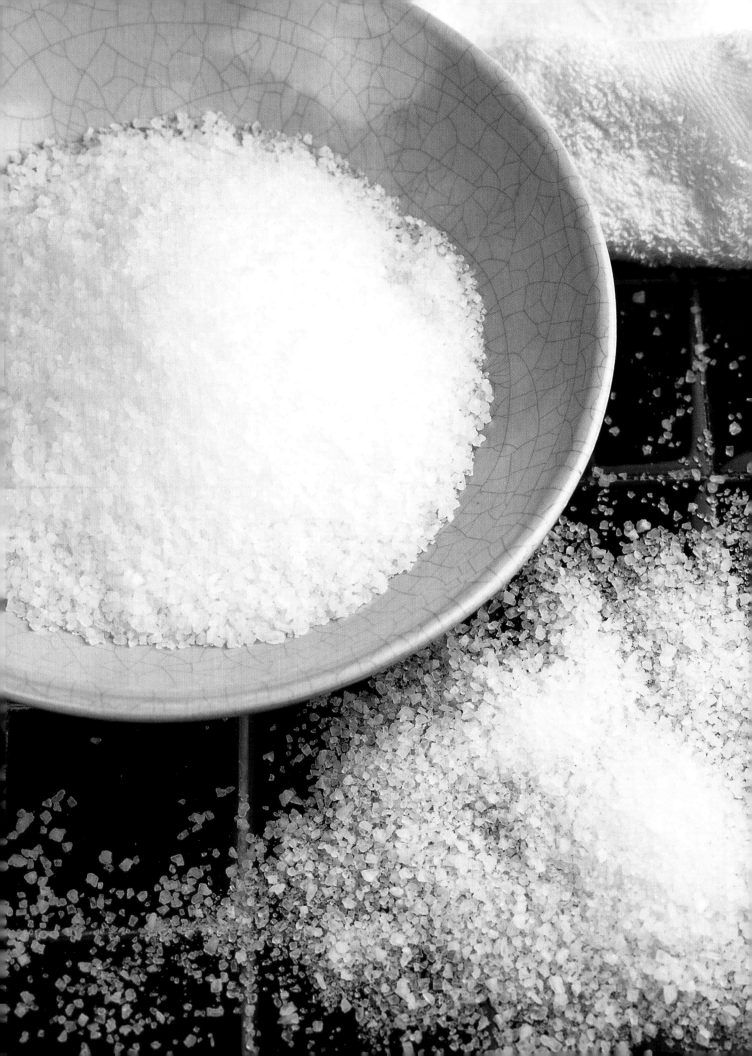

These **wonderful** bath salts have a delicious feminine aroma but needn't be exclusively for women. Why not share the bath!

Ylang ylang essential oil is wonderfully **relaxing** and is reputed to be an aphrodisiac; certainly it is difficult not to feel sexy after smelling its alluring, exotic sweetness. Bergamot is the perfect companion to ylang ylang because its sharp **citrus** aroma counteracts any heaviness and its stimulant properties give you the energy to put all those **sexy** thoughts to good use. Say no more!

BACCHANALIAN BATH SALTS

Ingredients
1 tsp sweet almond oil

6 drops bergamot essential oil

3 drops ylang ylang essential oil

4 oz Dead Sea salt

Equipment
Mixing bowl

Spoon

Dark or clear glass jars with lids

Method

1 Mix together the sweet almond oil and the essential oils, then stir in the Dead Sea salt. Pour into dark glass jars with lids or keep clear glass jars in a dark place to preserve the essential oils.

2 Add one heaped teaspoonful to the bath and enjoy.

Matching massage oil
You can also make a companion massage oil to gently smooth on after your bath and give a truly luxurious feeling. Mix the same amount of essential oils into 4 fl oz sweet almond oil. Pour into a dark glass bottle or store in clear glass in a dark place. Use after a bath or as a general body moisturizer.

Safety consideration
Bergamot essential oil makes the skin more sensitive to sunlight, so do not use it before exposing your skin to the sun.

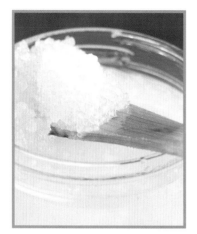

BEAUTIFUL BODY SCRUB

Ingredients

9 oz Dead Sea salt

4 fl oz sweet almond oil

1 tsp rosehip oil

3 drops lime essential oil

3 drops sweet orange essential oil

2 drops frankincense essential oil

1 drop clary sage essential oil

1 drop may chang essential oil

1 drop geranium essential oil

Equipment

Mixing bowl

Spoon

Dark or clear glass jars with tight-fitting lids

Method

1 Combine all the ingredients in a mixing bowl and stir well. Spoon the scrub into jars. Keep clear glass jars in a dark place to protect the essential oils from light.

2 Take a handful of the salt scrub and gently work it all over the body before rinsing off in a warm shower or bath, without using soap. Pat the skin dry with a soft towel and you will gain the full benefit of the oils, without any greasiness, and your skin will retain their delicate aroma.

Skin smoother

If you want to be really overindulgent, add about a teaspoon of calendula oil to the mix. Calendula is renowned for its skin-smoothing properties and is one of the best all-around skin remedies.

There's nothing quite like an exfoliating scrub to leave your skin silky and smooth.

This exfoliating scrub features the perfect mixture of essential oils to condition and

soothe, deodorize and pamper, while the sweet almond and rosehip oils are readily

absorbed and will nourish the skin. The Dead Sea salt can be replaced with Maldon salt

flakes to make a gentler scrub for sensitive skin.

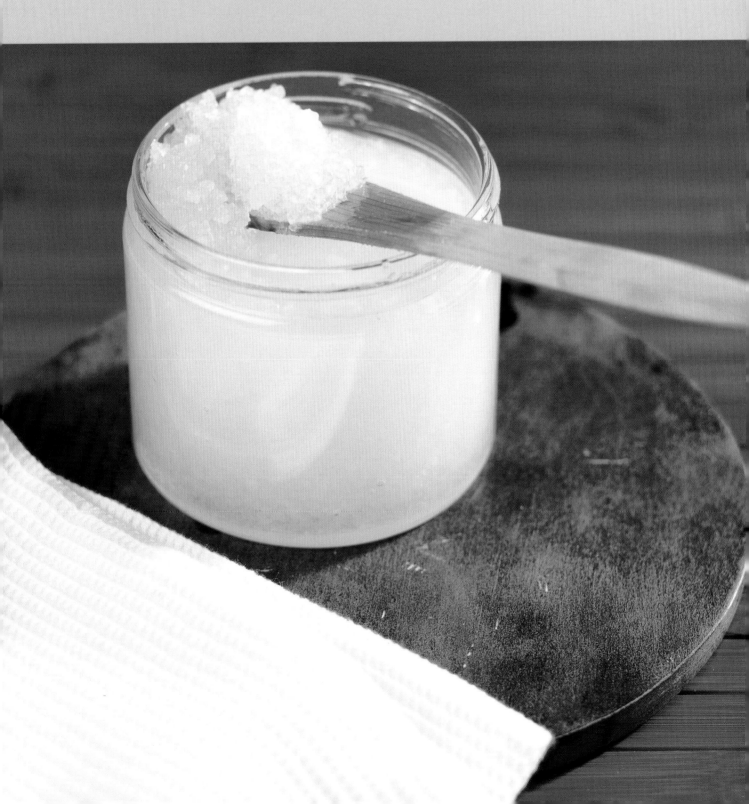

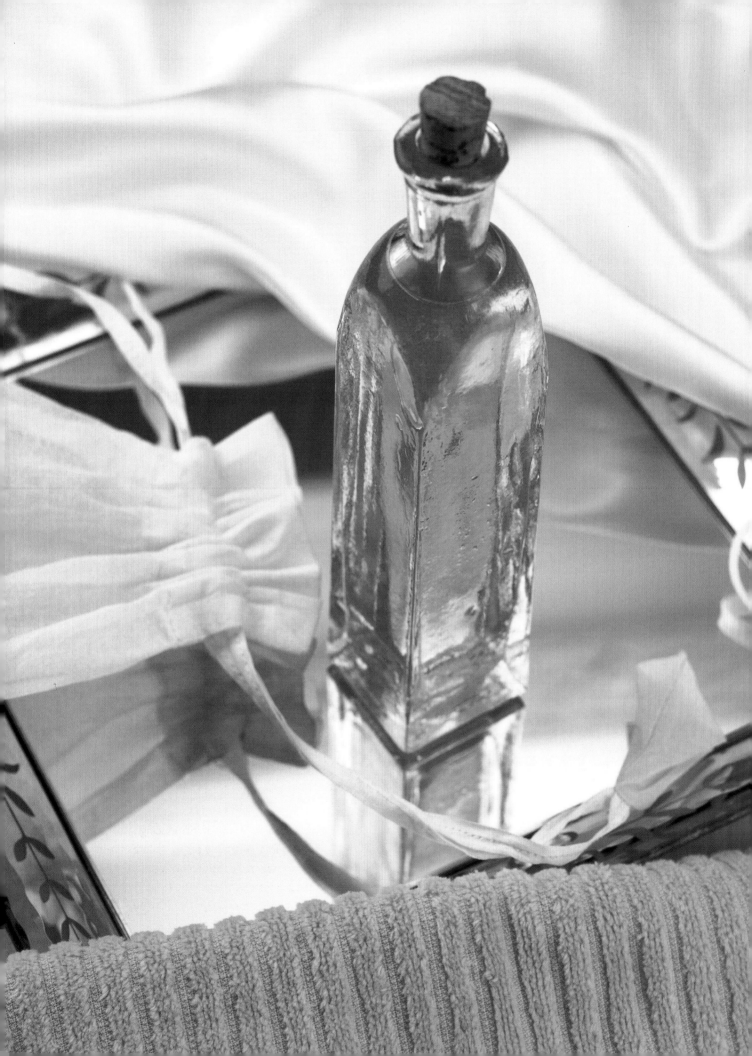

On a recent trip to Istanbul, I (Ada) took my daughter to an ancient but fully functional Turkish bath. The time and ritual involved in thoroughly cleansing the body, followed by a full massage—given by men and women who looked like wrestlers but had hands that were **gentle** and practiced—**impressed** me beyond words. Even my daughter, who is very prudish, asked me the next day if we could repeat this experience.

That massage could only be complemented by using this ultra-feminine oil, which takes into consideration the whole person: mind, body, and spirit.

Ylang ylang has a **calming** and relaxing effect, and maybe this is the reason it is considered an aphrodisiac. Clary sage can be described as both **euphoric** and **relaxing**.

VENUS MASSAGE OIL

Ingredients
4 fl oz sweet almond oil

1 tsp ylang ylang essential oil

1 tsp clary sage essential oil

Equipment
Dark or clear glass bottle with lid

Method
1 Mix the sweet almond oil with the essential oils in a glass bottle. Store a clear glass bottle in a dark place to preserve the essential oils.

2 Let your partner massage the oil in all over.

The benefits of massage
Massage provides us with the most effective way of introducing essential oils to the body. The skin, our largest body organ, absorbs these oils, and when the whole body is massaged a considerable amount of essential oil can be taken into the bloodstream in a short time. The therapeutic benefits are quickly felt and the whole body is surrounded with the most delicious aroma.

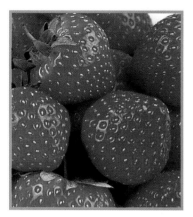

Masks are particularly effective for **clearing** up blemishes and refining open pores and coarse skin. They also **nourish**, heal, and soothe, as well as **exfoliate** the epidermis. But don't neglect the rest of your body. Dry elbows, knees, heels, and throats will all **benefit** greatly from a mask.

HOME ALONE FACE MASKS

Citrus fruits are toning and antiseptic for all skin types, while strawberries soften and combat oiliness in normal or combination skin. Tropical fruits, such as pineapple and figs, are excellent exfoliants, without any scratchy bits. We normally choose organic fruits, which should be mashed and drained of any juices.

USING MASKS

Ideally, masks should be used on a face that has been deeply cleansed, and they should be applied to slightly damp skin, avoiding contact with the eyes. They should be left on for 10 to 30 minutes—the individual recipes have their own suggested times—while you relax in a supine position. Make the most of this pleasurable experience by placing a pillow under your knees as well as one under your head and listening to your favorite music.

Rinse the mask off with lukewarm water or, even better, make an herbal infusion of lavatera, chamomile, or lime tree leaves; let cool to body temperature and strain it (see page 20); then take off the mask by gently splashing the infusion over the skin.

Leave the face to dry naturally or gently pat dry with a soft towel.

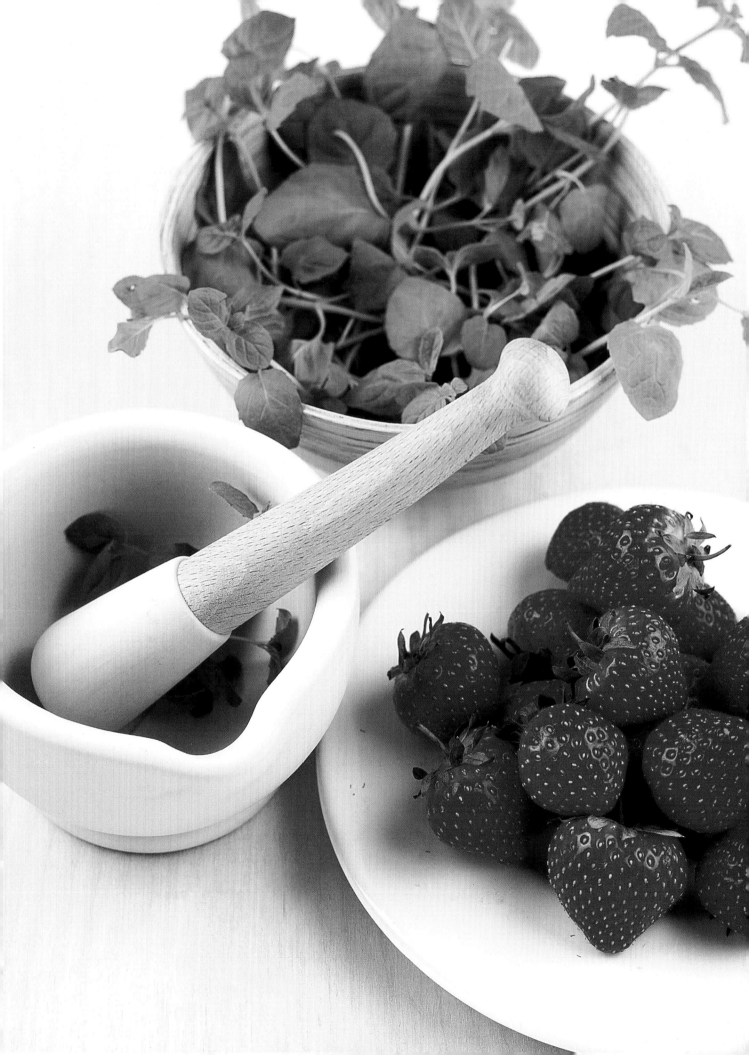

MASK FOR DRY SKIN

Honey is processed by bees from the nectar of flowers and has a natural quality that enhances its

healing properties. It is very good for skin in need of moisture. Almonds soften and smooth the skin,

while apricots and peaches refine coarse skin.

Ingredients

2 ripe apricots or 1 ripe peach

2 Tbsp honey

2 heaped Tbsp ground almonds

Equipment

Sharp knife

Fork

Mixing bowl

Method

1 Peel, pit, and mash the apricots or peach. Drain away any juice and then mix the mashed fruit with the honey and almonds.

2 Apply the mask to thoroughly cleansed skin, avoiding the eye area. Leave on for 20 to 30 minutes and rinse with lukewarm water or an infusion of lavatera or chamomile flowers.

MASK FOR OILY SKIN

With the tonic, astringent properties of lemons and the moisturizing and nourishing benefits of grapes,

pear, and egg white, which tightens the skin, this face mask is one of our favorites. You can also

use it for combination skin on the appropriate areas.

Ingredients

1 egg white

Handful seedless green grapes or
1 large ripe pear

Juice of half a lemon

1 tsp bran

18 fl oz mineral water

10 drops witch hazel

Equipment

Mixing bowl

Fork

Sharp knife

Method

1 Beat the egg white until it forms soft white peaks, then peel and mash the grapes or pear, draining away any juice.

2 Mix the egg white with the lemon juice, bran, and fruits. The mixture should be light and fluffy.

3 Gently massage this mask into the skin, paying particular attention to the nose, chin, and forehead and avoiding the delicate eye area. Leave it on for about 15 minutes. Mix the mineral water and witch hazel and use it to rinse off the mask.

MASK FOR NORMAL SKIN

This mask is almost good enough to eat—the smell of strawberries makes it irresistible.

The wheat germ oil is full of vitamin E for moisture and healing.

Ingredients

5–6 large, ripe strawberries

A handful of spearmint leaves

1 tsp wheat germ oil

1 tsp orange juice

Equipment

Blender

Method

1 Liquidize the strawberries and spearmint leaves, then add the wheat germ oil and orange juice.

2 Spread the mixture evenly on the face. For a complete summer feeling, put two thin slices of peeled cucumber over your eyelids, then relax for 20 to 30 minutes. Rinse the mask off with lukewarm water or an infusion of lime tree leaves.

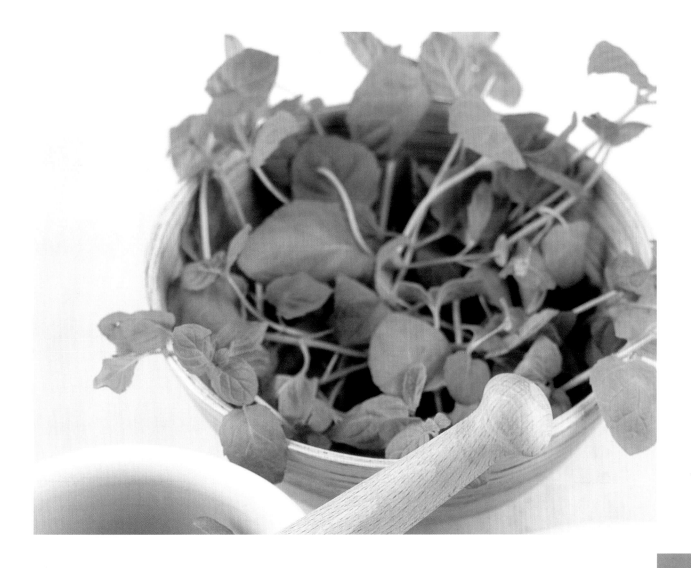

Nails show your state of health just as clearly as the condition of your skin, eyes, or hair. So use this cream once a week to hide any secrets your hands may want to tell.

Lemon essential oil is great for treating brittle nails and has a brightening effect on the skin. Myrrh essential oil will help any fungal infection and is invaluable for healing chapped, irritated skin. Myrrh is reputed to have been carried by the Ancient Greeks as they went into battle, because of its strong antiseptic and wound-healing properties. So it should have no problem remedying torn cuticles.

REALLY CUTE CUTICLE CREAM

Ingredients
2½ fl oz mineral water

2 handfuls of young nettle tops

3½ oz cocoa butter

¾ oz glycerine

1 tsp lemon essential oil

½ tsp myrrh essential oil

Equipment
Measuring jug

Sieve

Stainless-steel saucepan

Wooden spoon

Dark or clear glass jars with tight-fitting lids

Method

1 Infuse the nettle tops in boiling mineral water for 10 minutes (see page 20). Strain and allow to cool.

2 Melt the cocoa butter in a stainless-steel saucepan over low heat. Beat in the glycerine with a wooden spoon and slowly add the nettle infusion, stirring continuously.

3 Allow the cream to cool to body temperature and add the essential oils. Spoon into airtight jars and shake until the lotion has cooled completely, to stop the oil and water from separating. Keep clear glass containers in a dark place to ensure the essential oils are well preserved.

4 Once a week, soak your hands in a warm infusion of lavatera and chamomile flowers. Take an orange stick with a cotton pad on the end and gently push back the cuticles. Then massage the nails with the Really Cute Cuticle Cream.

> **Safety consideration**
> Do not use myrrh while pregnant. For this recipe, substitute lavender essential oil.

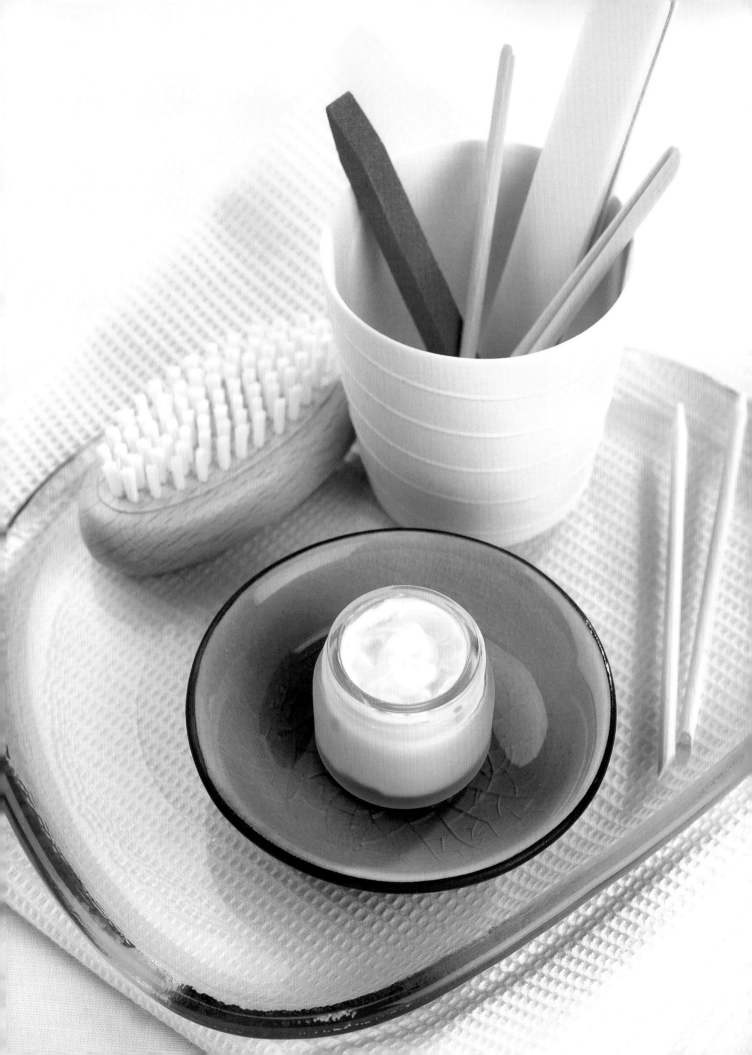

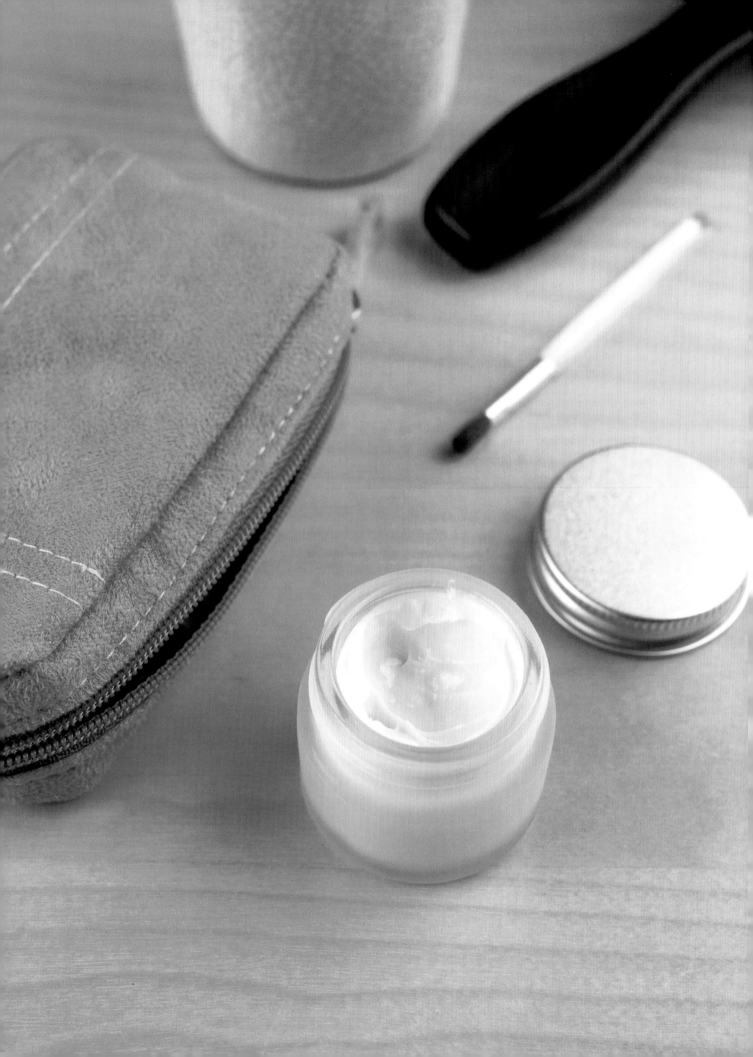

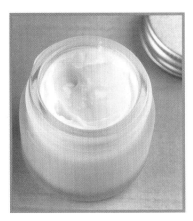

Dry, chapped lips can be a nightmare, especially in the cold winter months, and mean that you won't be in the right frame of mind for kissing! Keep this lip salve with you at all times and pucker up!

KISS "N" TELL LIP SALVE

Ingredients

1 oz beeswax

2 Tbsp sweet almond oil

2 Tbsp calendula oil

3 drops lavender essential oil

Equipment

Stainless-steel saucepan

Wooden spoon

Small glass jar with lid

Method

1 Melt the almond and calendula oils and the beeswax together in a stainless-steel saucepan over low heat, stirring continuously.

2 When the beeswax has completely melted, remove from the heat and continue to stir until the mixture cools to body temperature.

3 Add the lavender oil and stir thoroughly. If you wish, you can add another essential oil to complement the lavender.

4 Transfer the mixture to a small glass jar and leave to set until cool.

GIFTWRAPPING IDEAS

The recipes in this chapter make perfect presents—who wouldn't appreciate a gorgeously

wrapped pampering beauty product? Try putting one or two items in a gift box with some

shredded tissue paper or use sheer fabrics and shiny ribbons to add that special touch. A

handmade label in the shape of a heart is perfect for a bottle of Venus massage oil!

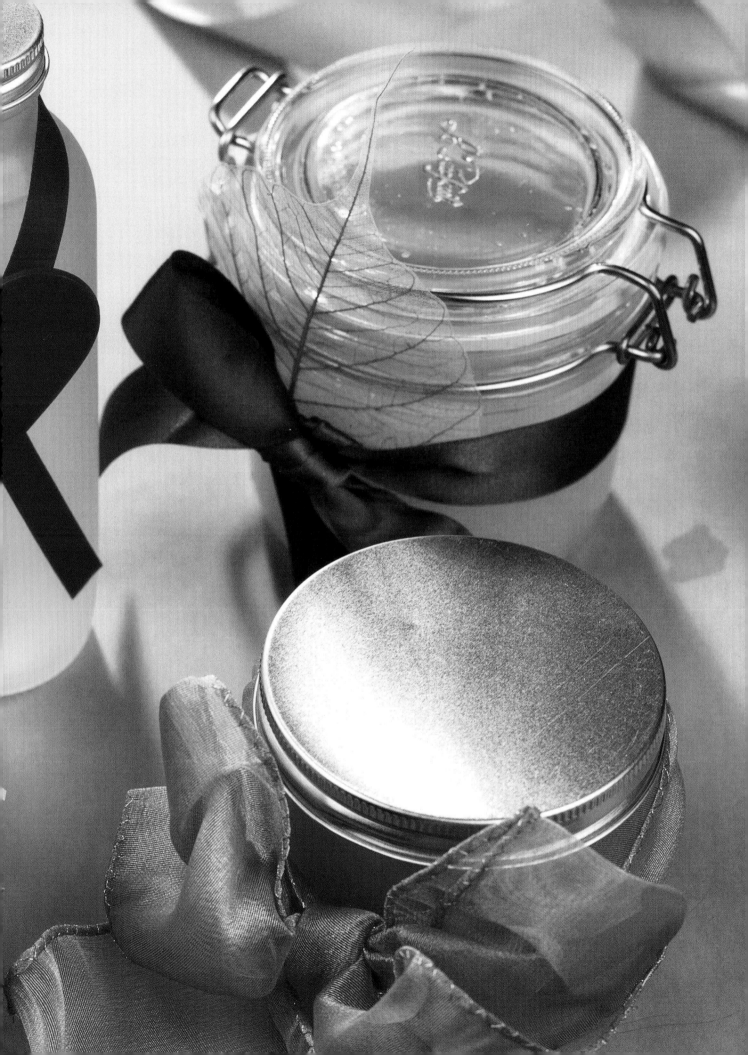

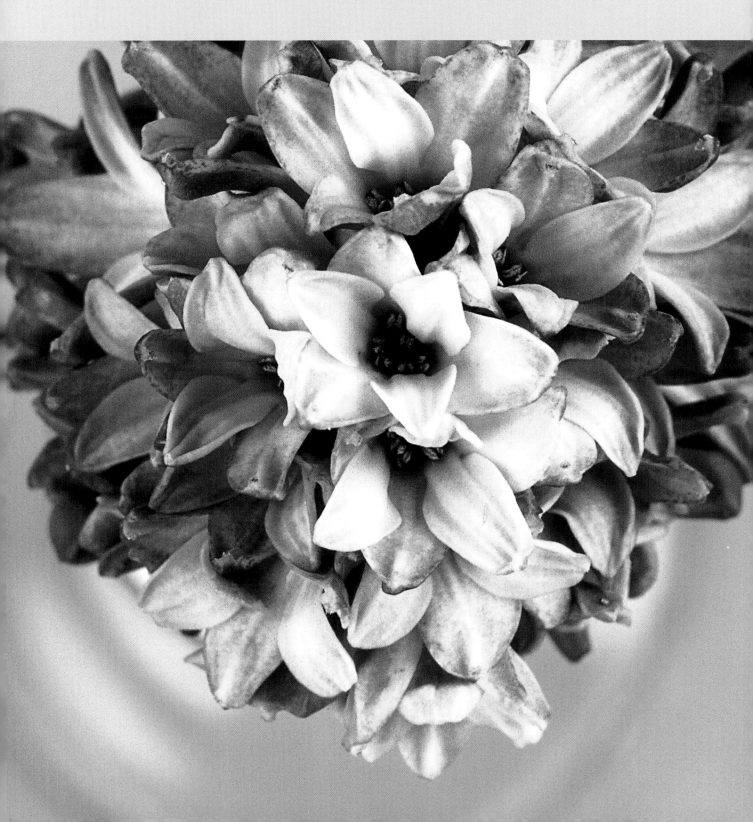

RELAX & REBALANCE

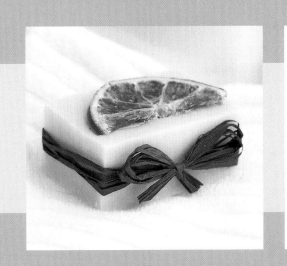 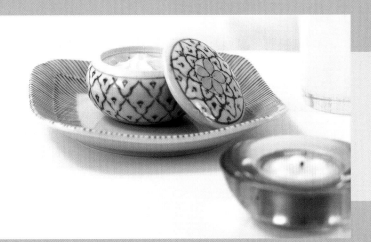

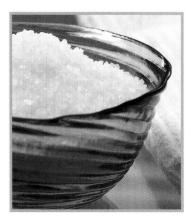

Here we have combined **elderflowers** with two of the most **fragrant** essential oils, plus mineralized Dead Sea **salts** and rosehip oil to **pamper** the skin. It only takes a few minutes to put together this recipe.

HEARTS-AND-FLOWERS BATH SALTS

Ingredients

1 tsp rosehip oil

6 drops lime essential oil

3 drops geranium essential oil

4 oz Dead Sea salt

A head of dried elderflowers

Equipment

Mixing bowl

Spoon

Dark or clear glass jars with lids

Method

1 Mix together the rosehip oil and the essential oils, then stir in the Dead Sea salt and elderflowers. Spoon into glass jars with lids, or keep clear glass jars in a dark place to protect the essential oils from light.

2 Add a teaspoonful to the bath. These salts are better used when freshly made, so store them for only a month or so for optimum results.

Elderflowers

Elderflowers are one of the beauties of the countryside, heralding the spring with their fresh, delicate aroma and dainty lace flowerheads. When dried, the flowers can be used to make a refreshing tea. Elder has a long history of use in creams and ointments. The flowers can be infused and added to creams for use on hands and body, or a few fresh flowers mixed with live yogurt makes a great face mask to clear the skin and prevent wrinkles.

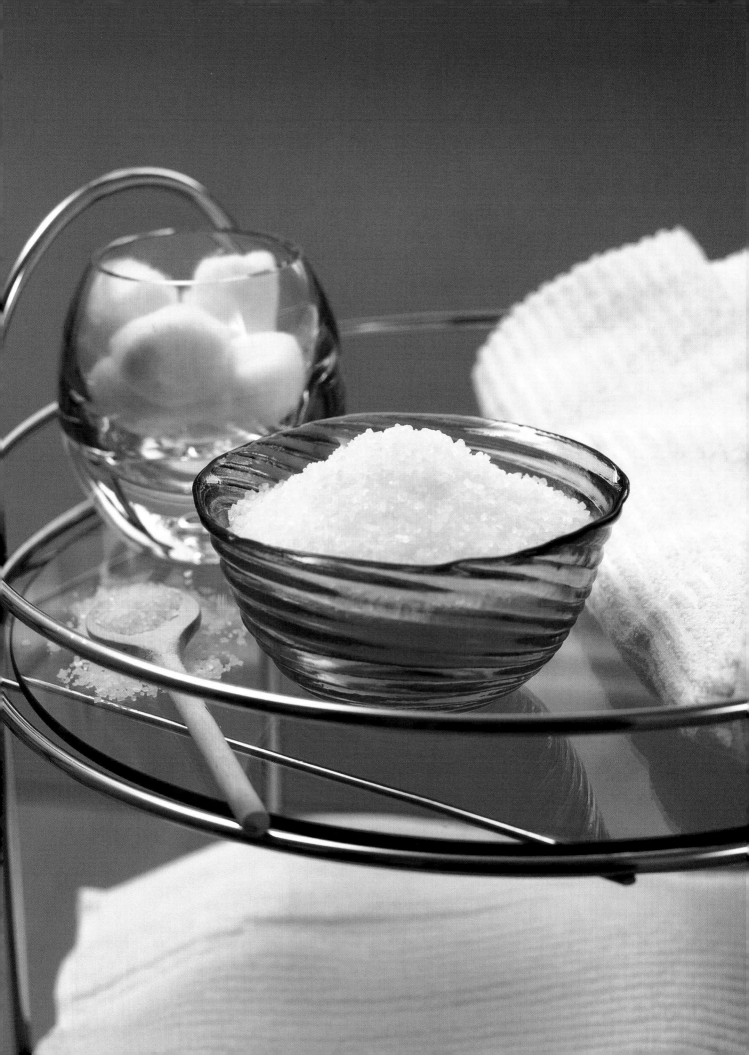

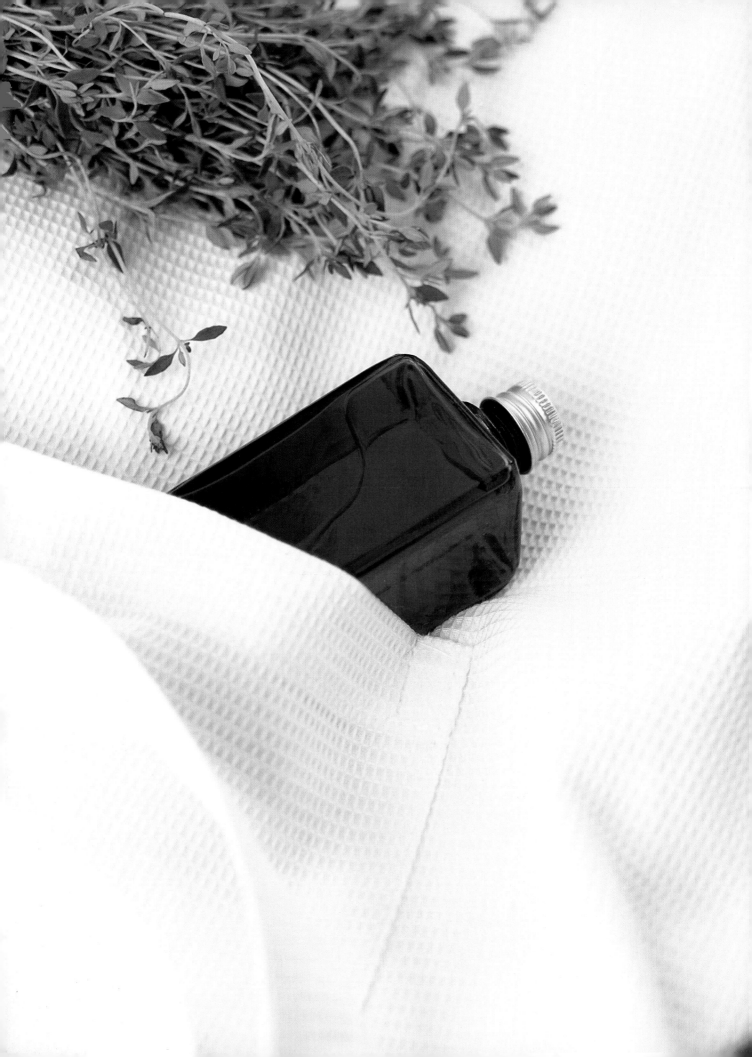

This **therapeutic** massage oil induces deep sleep and eases the aches and pains of the day. Thyme is an amazing essential oil because it is used to stimulate circulation, **ease** fatigue, and **soothe** rheumatic pains, and it is one of the best oils to use for insomnia because of its **balancing** effect on the nervous system. Combined with sweet orange essential oil, which has sedative properties, and juniper berry essential oil, which will **detoxify** the body overnight, you'll be asleep before the massage ends.

THYMELESS SLEEP OIL

Ingredients

4 fl oz sweet almond oil

8 drops thyme essential oil

8 drops sweet orange essential oil

4 drops juniper berry essential oil

Equipment

Dark or clear glass bottle with tight-fitting lid

Method

1 Mix all the oils together in a dark bottle with a tight-fitting lid, or store a clear bottle in the dark to preserve the oils.

2 Use as a massage oil before bed. Even a little rubbed into the hands and arms will help you sleep.

Safety considerations

Avoid juniper berry and thyme essential oils while pregnant. For this recipe, use lavender instead.

If you suffer from nut allergies, you should replace the sweet almond oil with grapeseed or sunflower oil.

While most men do not have a specific facial-cleansing routine, we think they'll **love** this soap with

exfoliating properties to unblock pores and deep-cleanse skin, leaving the face moisturized and smooth.

The aroma of "Boy, Oh Boy" is fruity but manly, with a deep undertone of cinnamon spice. A **warming**,

stimulating essential oil, cinnamon is ideal for a masculine soap when combined with citrus aromas. Grapefruit

and sweet orange essential oils have been added for their "**sunshine**" aromas that lift the spirits and soothe

the skin. Sprinkle poppy seeds in the finished soap to give gentle exfoliation and an interesting texture.

"BOY, OH BOY" SCRUB SOAP FOR MEN

Ingredients

6 fl oz sunflower oil

6 fl oz olive oil

5 oz coconut oil

2$\frac{1}{2}$ oz caustic soda

8 fl oz mineral water

2 tsp grapefruit essential oil

1 tsp sweet orange essential oil

1 tsp cinnamon leaf essential oil

2 Tbsp poppy seeds

Equipment

General equipment (see page 12)

Safety equipment (see page 13)

Wooden board

Tray

Method

1 Work in a well-ventilated area. Oil and line a plastic mold with waxed paper.

2 Melt the sunflower, olive, and coconut oils in a large, heavy-based stainless-steel saucepan over low heat.

3 Wearing protective goggles, a mask, an apron, and long rubber gloves, add the caustic soda to the mineral water in a tall plastic bucket and stir with a plastic spatula until dissolved.

4 Using one jam thermometer for the oils and another for the caustic soda mixture (lye water), allow both temperatures to reach 96°F—you may need to reheat the oils. Wearing protective clothing, immediately pour the lye water into the oils, off the heat. Combine the mixtures thoroughly using the spatula. Continuously stir for approximately 15 minutes.

5 Tracing occurs when a drizzle of the mixture on the surface of the soap leaves a visible line. At this point, add the essential oils and poppy seeds and combine thoroughly. Pour into the prepared mold and place in a safe, warm, dry place for 24 hours, covering with cardboard to keep the heat in.

6 Wearing protective gloves, turn out the soap onto a wooden board covered with waxed paper. Peel off the lining paper and cut the soap into the desired shapes using a carving knife or cookie cutters. If the mixture is too soft to cut, leave for another 24 hours. Space out the cut soaps on a tray lined with waxed paper and leave in a dark, warm, dry place for four weeks, turning several times during the maturing process.

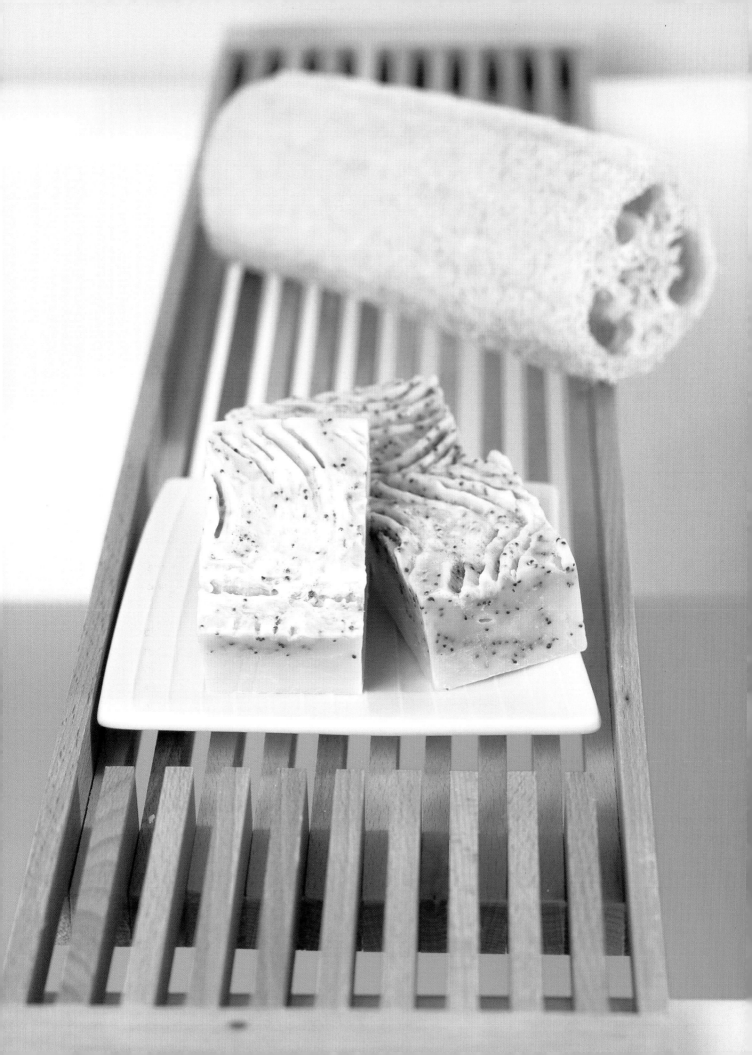

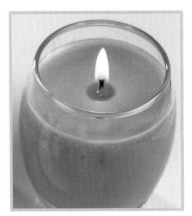

This **dreamy**, creamy lotion to stroke all over is enriching for both your physical and psychological self. Your **body** will be eternally grateful for its **moisture** treat and the combination of two **superrelaxing** essential oils.

DREAMBOAT ALL-OVER NIGHT CREAM

Ingredients

1/2 oz beeswax

1/2 oz cocoa butter

2 oz coconut oil

2 Tbsp sweet almond oil

4 Tbsp mineral water

1 tsp lavender essential oil

1 tsp ylang ylang essential oil

Equipment

Stainless-steel saucepan

Wooden spoon

Dark or clear glass jar with lid

Method

1 Place the beeswax, cocoa butter, coconut oil, and sweet almond oil in a large, heavy-based stainless-steel saucepan and melt slowly over low heat. Beat the mineral water in vigorously with a wooden spoon.

2 Take the pan off the heat and keep stirring until the cream has cooled to body temperature. Add the essential oils and mix thoroughly. Pour into airtight jars and shake until cool to prevent the water and oil from separating. Keep clear jars in a dark place to preserve the essential oils.

3 Rub the cream in all over the body as part of your bedtime routine—and look forward to golden dreams.

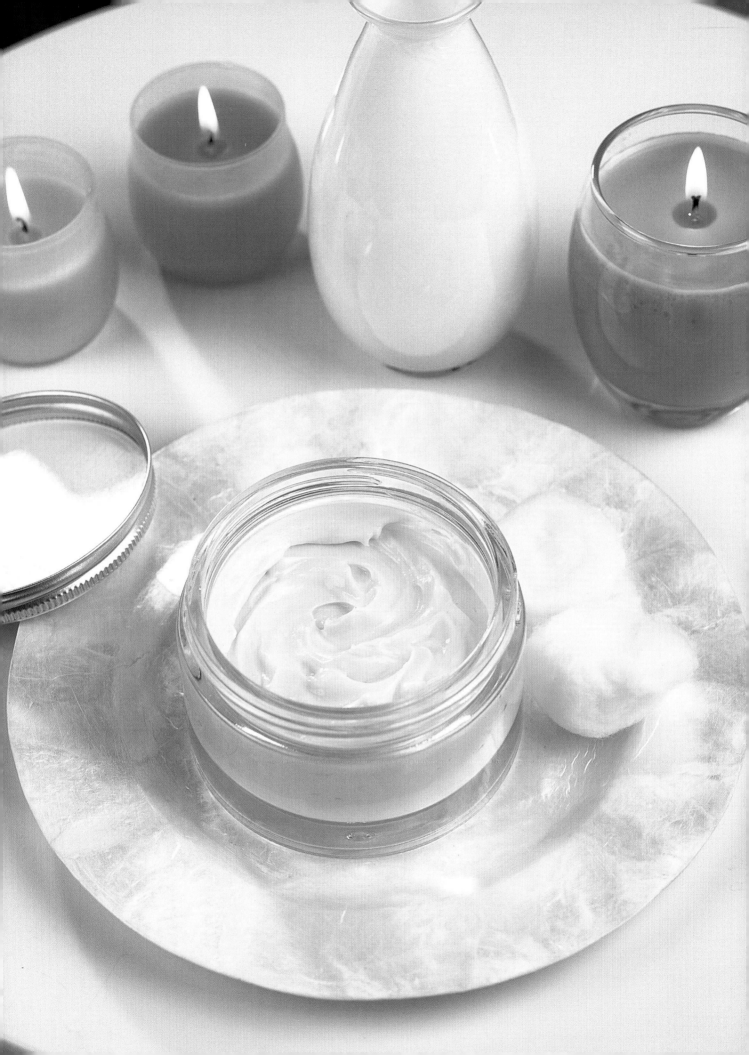

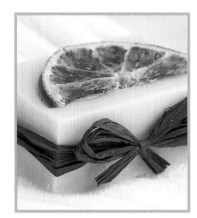

TANGERINE DREAM SOAP

Ingredients

10 fl oz extra-virgin olive oil

4 fl oz sweet almond oil

2$\frac{1}{2}$ oz coconut oil

2$\frac{1}{2}$ oz palm oil

1$\frac{1}{2}$ oz beeswax

2$\frac{1}{2}$ oz caustic soda

8 fl oz mineral water

2 tsp tangerine essential oil

1 tsp sweet orange essential oil

1 tsp lavender essential oil

Equipment

General equipment (see page 12)

Safety equipment (see page 13)

Wooden board

Tray

Method

1 Work in a well-ventilated area. Oil and line a plastic mold with waxed paper.

2 Melt the olive, sweet almond, coconut, and palm oils with the beeswax in a large, heavy-based stainless-steel saucepan over low heat.

3 Wearing protective eyewear, a face mask, an apron, and long rubber gloves, pour the caustic soda into the mineral water in a tall plastic bucket and stir with a plastic spatula until completely dissolved.

4 Using two jam thermometers, one for the oils and one for the caustic soda mixture (lye water), monitor both solutions until they equalize at 131°F. At this point, while still wearing the protective clothing, pour the lye water into the oils and stir thoroughly, continuing to stir until the mixture traces—when a drizzle of mixture leaves a line on the surface of the soap.

5 Pour in the essential oils and mix thoroughly, then pour the soap into the prepared mold. Cover with cardboard and leave in a safe, warm, dry place for 24 hours.

6 Wearing gloves—the soap is still caustic at this stage—turn out the soap onto a board lined with waxed paper. Remove the lining paper and cut the soaps to the desired size with a carving knife. Space the soaps out on a tray covered with waxed paper and store for four weeks in a warm, dry place, turning occasionally.

7 Use this soap in a leisurely bath to really appreciate its magic.

Achieving a **balance** is what aromatherapy is all about, and it's what we would all love to have in our lives, too. This soap balances the wonderful **relaxing** and sedative powers of lavender and sweet orange with the fresh, lively aroma of tangerine essential oil. This is a **gentle**, unassuming soap with lashings of extra-virgin olive oil, sweet almond oil, and coconut oil to enhance your skin.

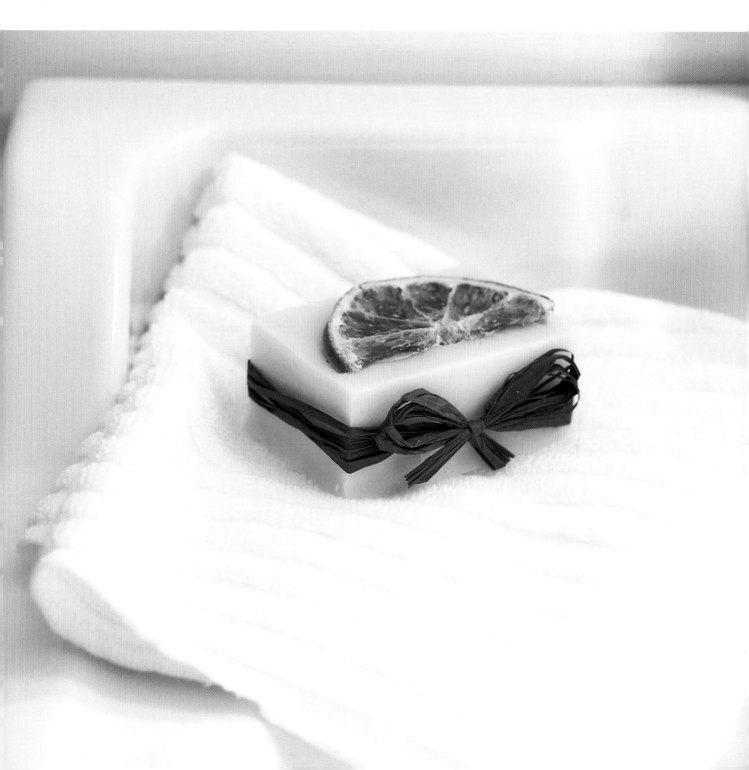

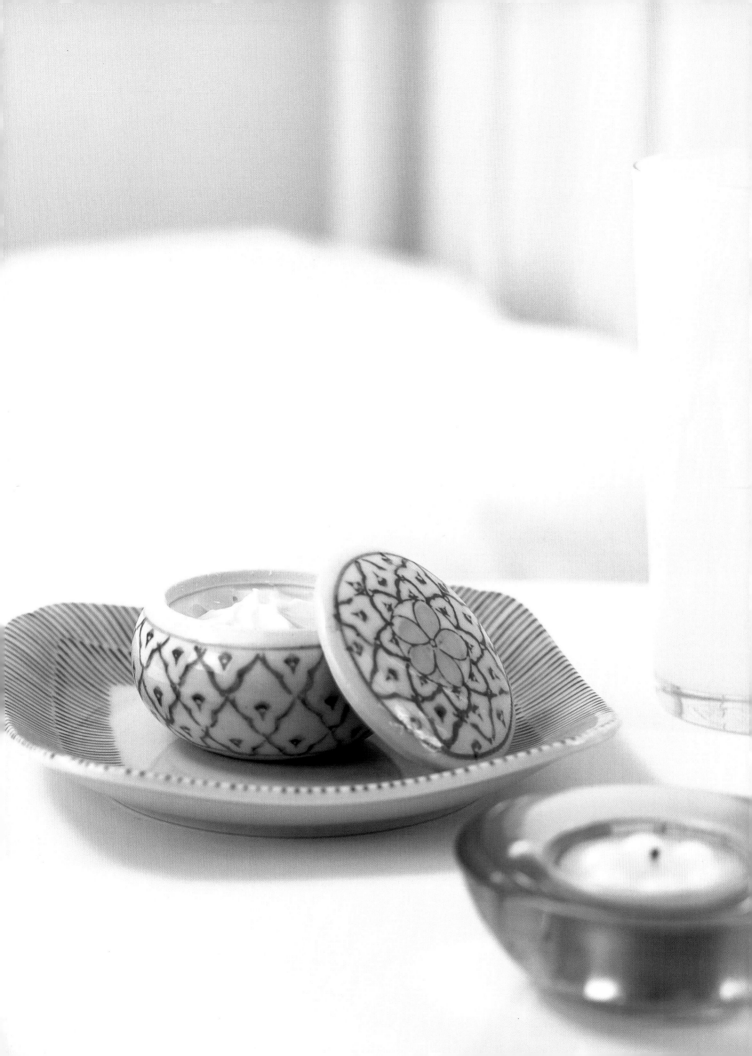

We have developed this face cream to tackle the effects of age on the skin. In skincare, **frankincense** is particularly helpful to older skin. It helps restore tone and slows down the appearance of wrinkles. It may even reduce the extent of wrinkles that have already formed. Lemon juice clears the complexion and, used in a face lotion, helps **banish wrinkles**, while lemon essential oil has a **brightening** effect on sallow skin and age spots, aids circulation, and has a mild bleaching effect. The calendula infusion will add to the **soothing** effect of this cream and is useful for combating dryness and flakiness.

MOONSHADOW FACIAL NIGHT CREAM

Ingredients

A handful of dried calendula flowers

3/4 oz beeswax

1 fl oz calendula oil

1 1/2 fl oz sweet almond oil

2 tsp lemon juice

1/2 tsp frankincense essential oil

1/4 tsp lemon essential oil

Equipment

Measuring jug

Sieve

Stainless-steel saucepan

Wooden spoon

Dark or clear glass jars with lids

Method

1. Make an herbal infusion with the calendula flowers and 10 fl oz boiling water (see page 20). Strain and set aside to cool.

2. Melt the beeswax in a large, heavy-based stainless-steel saucepan. Add the oils, beating steadily with a wooden spoon, then add 2 Tbsp of the calendula infusion and the lemon juice in a slow trickle.

3. Take the saucepan off the heat and continue to stir until the lotion has cooled to body temperature. Add the essential oils, then decant the cream into jars and shake until the lotion has completely cooled. If you are using clear glass jars, keep them in a dark place away from direct sunlight to preserve the essential oils.

4. Before bed, cleanse the face, then gently smooth on the night cream, working upward from jaw to cheekbones, around the eyes, and over the forehead. Work the cream into the neck from the base to the chin.

It is no accident that so many of the essential oils regarded as

antidepressants are the product of summer flowers, such as

lavender, jasmine, and geranium. At a deep, subconscious level, they

evoke **warm** breezes, **sunny** days, summer gardens, vacations, and

happy memories. Citrus oils, particularly bergamot, can also be

used to lift your mood if you are stressed or unhappy.

EMOTIONAL RESCUE MASSAGE OIL

Ingredients
4 fl oz sweet almond oil

1 tsp lavender essential oil

1 tsp bergamot essential oil

$\frac{1}{2}$ tsp lemongrass essential oil

Equipment
Plastic jug

Wooden spoon

Dark or clear glass bottle with tight-fitting lid

Method

1 Measure the sweet almond oil in a plastic cup, then add the essential oils, stirring continuously.

2 Pour the massage oil into a bottle and close the lid. Keep a clear glass bottle in a dark place to preserve the essential oils.

3 Immediately before use, gently shake the bottle to mix the oils well. Always apply light, relaxed hands when massaging, unless you are properly trained. A gentle massage is much more soothing, and if you are not an expert you can do real damage by being heavy-handed.

The benefits of massage
After a long, stressful week, heal and restore yourself by massaging Emotional Rescue Massage Oil into either side of the spine, then let your mind drift away to peace and calm. Massage almost always brings about muscular relaxation, even without the use of essential oils, though the combination of the two can have a dramatic effect.

Safety consideration
Bergamot essential oil should not be used on the skin before it is exposed to sunshine, since it makes the skin more sensitive to sunlight.

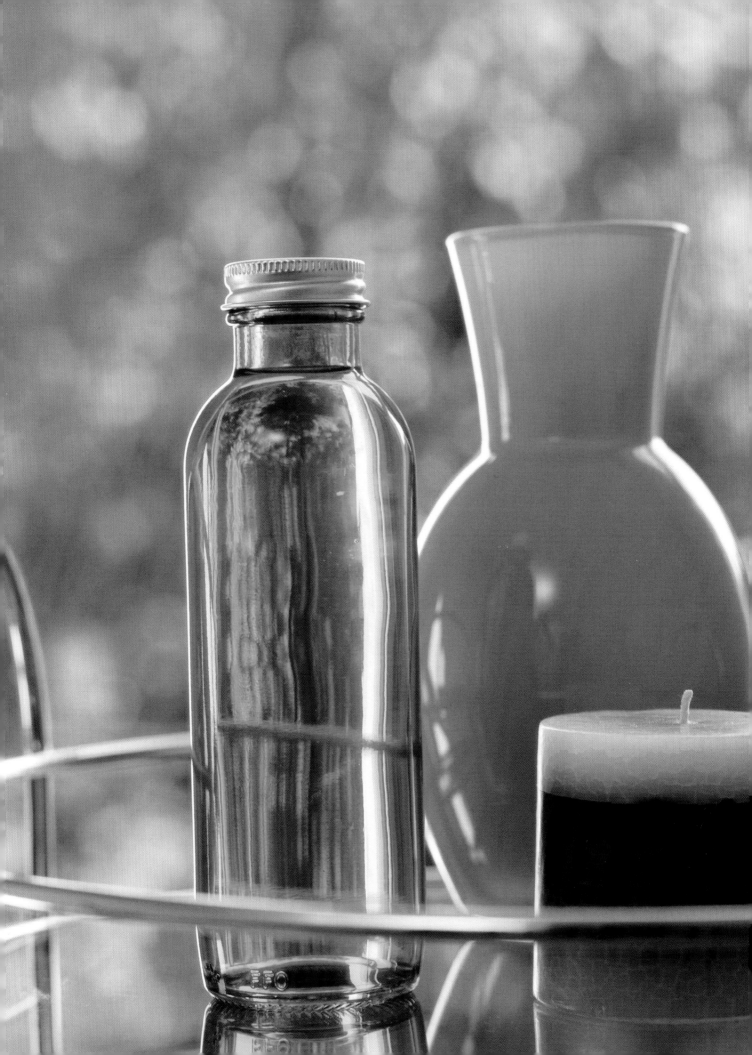

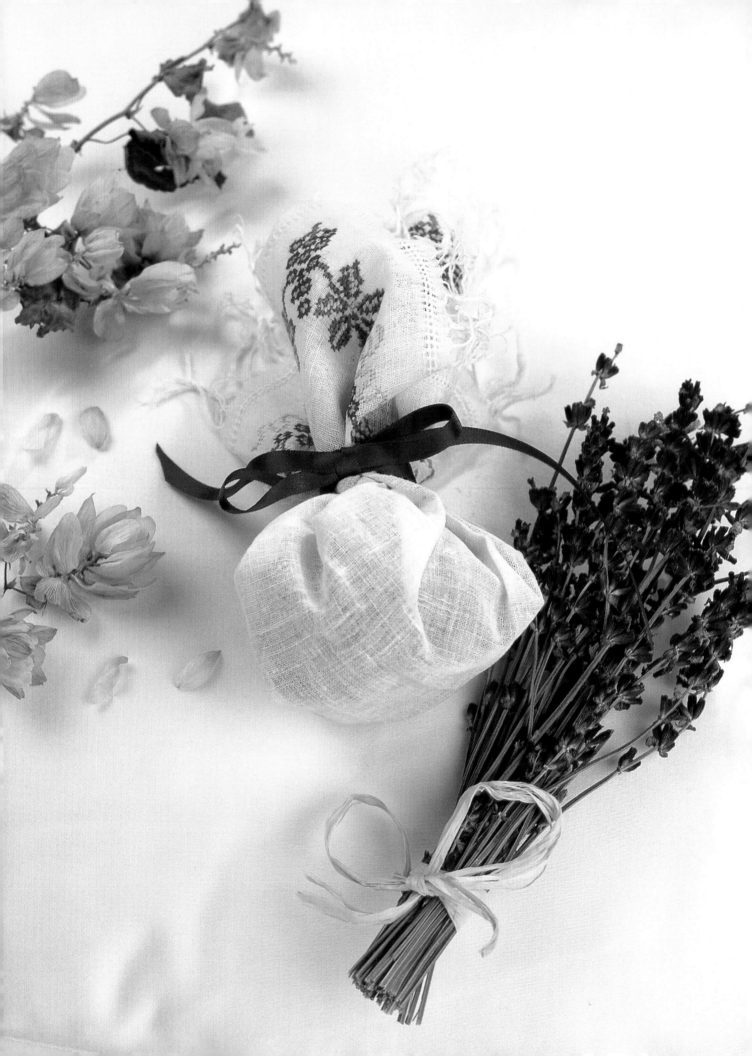

A small pouch filled with dried flowers can be placed inside your usual pillowcase to **relax** your mind and send you off to sleep. The **therapeutic benefits** of the plants used depend very much on the way they are gathered and dried. **Flowers** should be picked in dry weather, once the sun has risen and the dew has cleared. Leaves should be **gathered** before they are fully developed. To ensure the dried plants conserve their active ingredients at the highest level, they should be dried in the **sun**, a greenhouse, or an oven.

SWEET DREAMS HERBAL PILLOWS

Ingredients
Dried flowers: for a peaceful sleep try hops, cowslips, lemon balm, and lavender

Equipment
Muslin or a loose-woven fabric

Scissors

Ribbon

Method

1 Cut out a piece of fabric, approximately 8 inches square, and place the dried-flower mixture in the center. Gather up the edges of the fabric and tie a pretty ribbon around the neck of the pouch to hold the flowers in. Allow room for the dried plants to "breathe" and to release their therapeutic aromas.

2 Tuck a pouch in the corner of your pillowcase and drift away on a fragrant cloud.

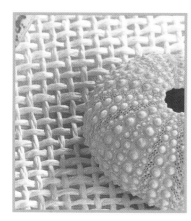

Just like a breath of **fresh** air, bracing and invigorating, this soap also has the wonderful scent of the **sea** (but without the fish!). We've added seaweed for texture and nutrients, sage essential oil for its antifungal properties, and petitgrain for the skin. Grapefruit essential oil **refreshes** and uplifts, while orange essential oil has a **calming** and balancing effect.

SEA AIR BODY SOAP

Ingredients

8 fl oz olive oil

1¹/₂ fl oz avocado oil

2 oz coconut oil

2 oz palm oil

1 oz beeswax

6¹/₂ fl oz mineral water

2 oz caustic soda

1¹/₂ tsp grapefruit essential oil

1 tsp sweet orange essential oil

¹/₂ tsp petitgrain essential oil

¹/₄ tsp sage essential oil

2 handfuls of arame seaweed

Equipment

General equipment (see page 12)

Safety equipment (see page 13)

Wooden board

Tray

Method

1 Work in a well-ventilated area. First oil and line a plastic mold with waxed paper.

2 Melt the olive oil, avocado oil, coconut oil, palm oil, and beeswax in a large heavy-based stainless-steel saucepan over low heat.

3 Using protective eyewear, an apron, and long rubber gloves, pour the caustic soda into the mineral water in a tall plastic bucket, stirring continuously with a plastic spatula to dissolve.

4 Using a separate thermometer for the oils and the caustic soda mixture (lye water), monitor both solutions until they reach 131°F. Still wearing the protective clothing, immediately pour the lye water into the oils and stir thoroughly. Continue stirring until "tracing" occurs (see page 11).

5 Add the essential oils, stirring well until they are thoroughly combined with the soap mixture, then do the same with the seaweed. Pour the soap into the prepared mold and make a "wave" pattern on the top of the soap using a spoon or a spatula. Leave to set for 24 hours, covered with cardboard in a warm, dry place.

6 Wearing protective gloves, turn the soap out onto a wooden board covered with waxed paper and cut, wave side up, into chunky bars. Space the bars out on a tray lined with waxed paper. Leave to cure in a warm, dry place for four weeks.

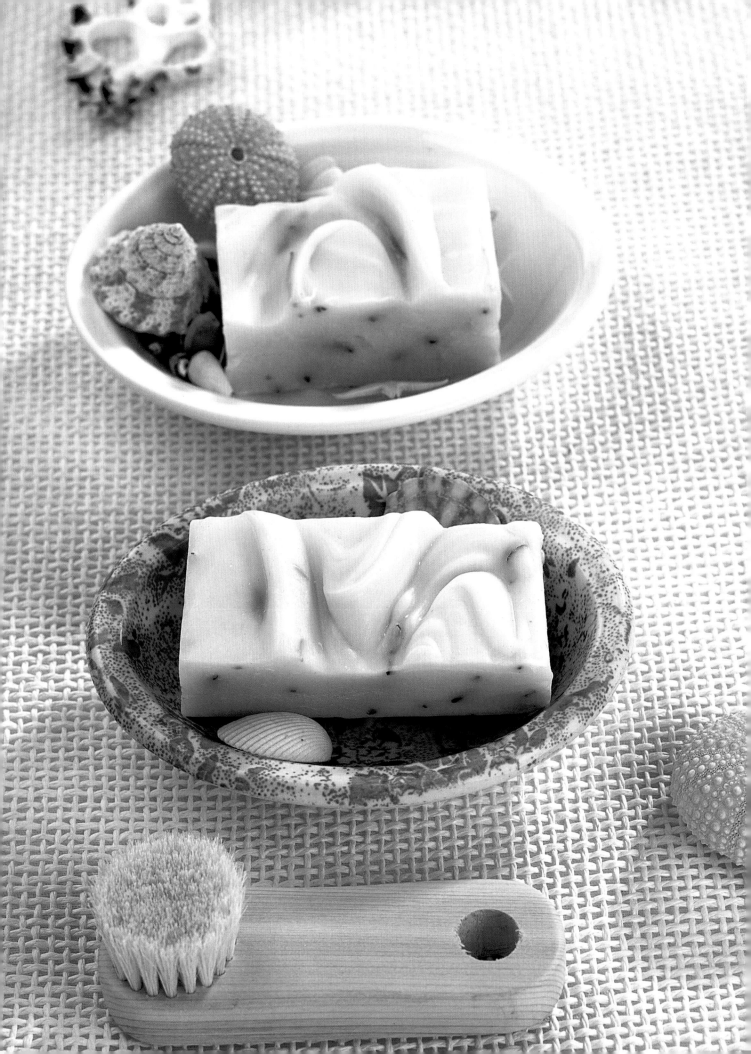

GIFTWRAPPING IDEAS

Blue, the color of the sea and the sky, is wonderfully calming and relaxing—perfect for wrapping up some of the soaps and other items in this chapter. A glass bottle wrapped in soft muslin and tied with a purple ribbon makes an elegant gift, while a smart checked ribbon smartens up a simple pot of face cream. For a special someone, place a handmade soap on a shell soap dish and tie with pretty blue ribbon.

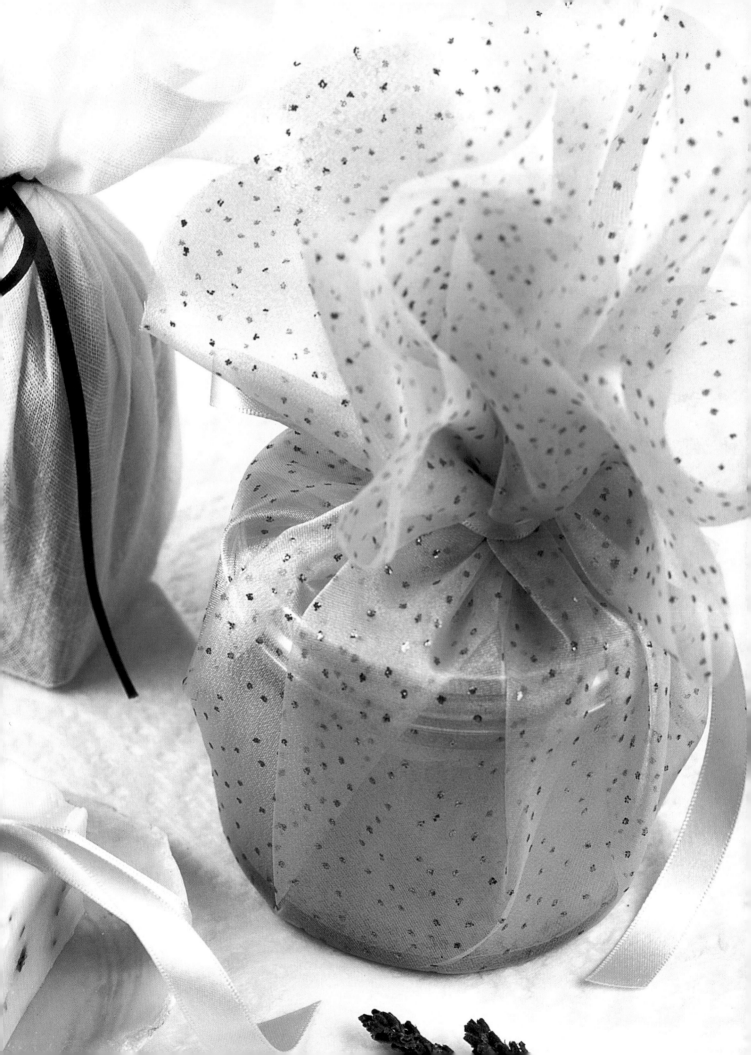

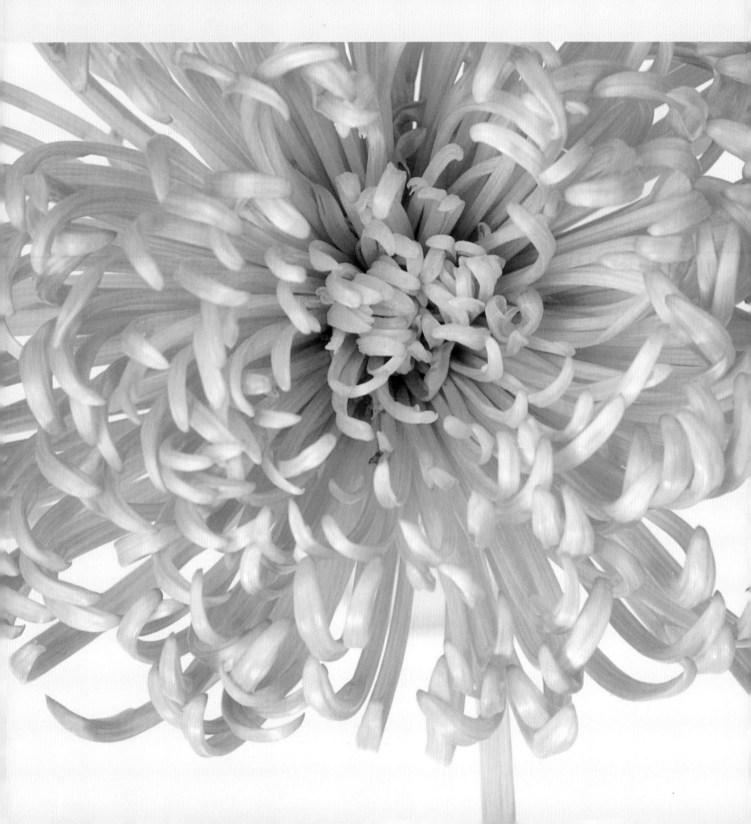

RESTORE & HEAL

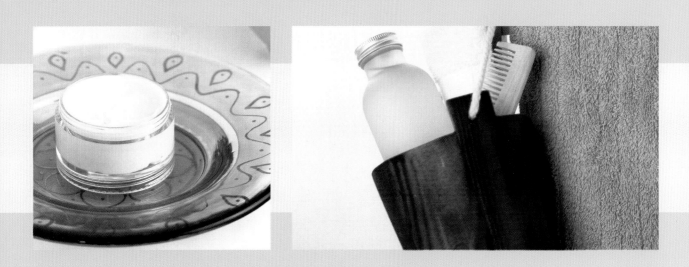

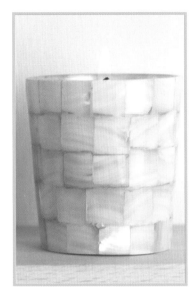

"Stop the world, I want to get off!" Whether it's you or a friend in crisis, this **delicious** mixture will help soothe troubled emotions and relieve some of the tension. Juniper berry is an **amazing** essential oil in that its cleansing, detoxifying properties work on the mind as well as the body, **reviving** the emotionally drained. Bergamot has the most delightful citrus aroma and immediately uplifts the spirits, making it the ideal companion for juniper berry. The result will leave you **refreshed**, lively, and ready for anything.

STOP THE WORLD DE-STRESS OIL

Ingredients
2 Tbsp sweet almond oil

8 drops bergamot essential oil

4 drops juniper berry essential oil

Equipment
Dark or clear glass bottle with tight-fitting lid

Method
1 Mix all the ingredients thoroughly in a bottle with a tight-fitting lid. Keep clear glass in the dark to preserve the essential oils.

2 Ideally, this oil should be used in conjunction with a wonderful massage, but if that isn't possible just smooth it onto arms, legs, hands, feet, or whatever part of the body is accessible at the time.

Safety considerations
Pregnant women, whom we hope won't be stressed, should in any case replace the juniper berry essential oil in this recipe with lavender.

Bergamot essential oil makes the skin more sensitive to sunlight, so do not use it if you are likely to be exposed to the sun.

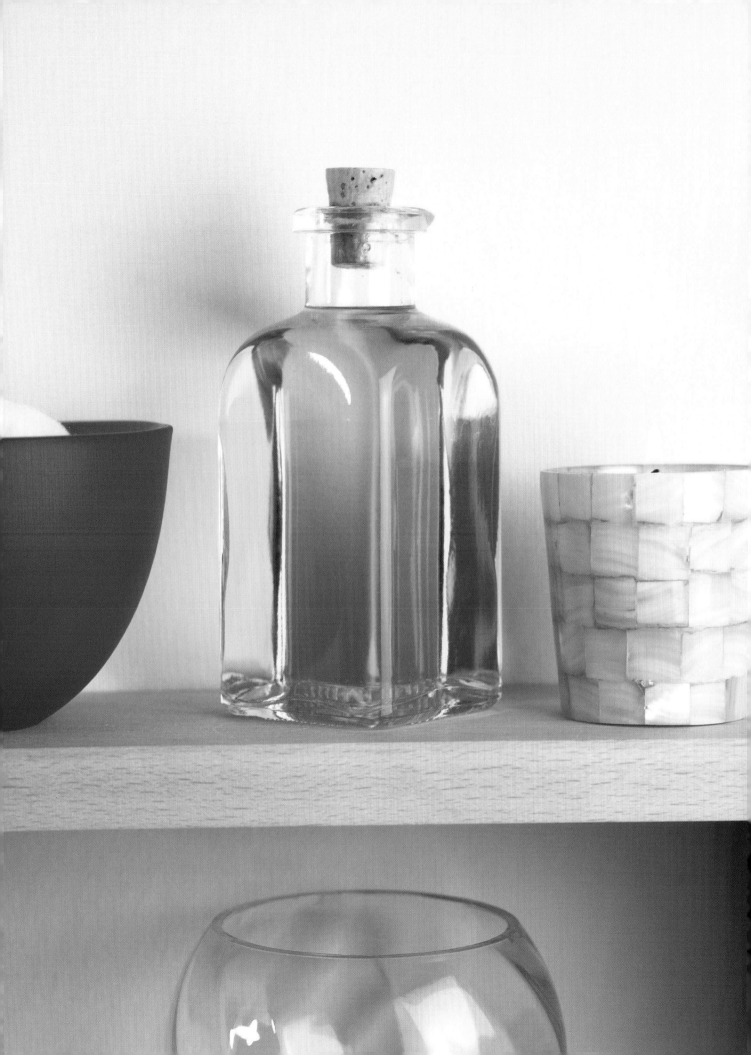

ANGEL HAIR THERAPEUTIC SHAMPOO BAR

Ingredients

9 fl oz mineral water

2 chamomile teabags

1¼ pints olive oil

3½ fl oz sweet almond oil

2 oz beeswax

2 oz coconut cream oil

4 oz caustic soda

4 tsp bergamot essential oil

2 tsp lavender essential oil

1 tsp geranium essential oil

1 tsp rosemary essential oil

Equipment

General equipment (see page 12)

Safety equipment (see page 13)

Sieve

Wooden board

Tray

Method

1 Boil the mineral water and pour over the chamomile teabags in a bowl. Leave to cool, then strain, reserving the infusion.

2 Work in a well-ventilated area. Oil and line a plastic mold with waxed paper.

3 Melt the olive and sweet almond oils with the beeswax and coconut cream oil in a stainless-steel saucepan over low heat, stirring regularly so that the coconut cream oil does not "catch" the bottom of the pan and burn.

4 Wearing protective gloves, goggles, a face mask, and an apron, pour the caustic soda into the chamomile infusion in a tall plastic bucket to make the lye water. Stir with a plastic spatula to dissolve.

5 Using one jam thermometer for the oils and one for the lye water, monitor both mixtures until they reach 131°F. Still wearing the protective clothing, immediately pour the lye water into the oils and mix thoroughly, stirring until tracing occurs—when a drizzle of the mixture makes a line on the surface of the soap.

6 Add the essential oils and mix well. Pour the soap into the prepared mold, cover with cardboard, and leave for 24 hours in a safe, warm, dry place.

7 The soap is still caustic at this stage, so wear protective gloves while you turn it out onto a wooden board covered with waxed paper. Peel off the lining paper and cut the bar into the desired shapes using a carving knife. Space the cut soaps out well on a tray covered with waxed paper and store in a dry, warm place for four weeks, turning occasionally to dry evenly.

> ### Recycling the teabags
> Save the chamomile teabags after you have made the infusion. They are great for soothing tired eyes when laid over the eyelids for five minutes.

We've come up with a combination that we think is the **ultimate** treatment for hair. This creamy, conditioning shampoo bar *revives* flagging (and thinning) locks and has a delectable aroma to boot! As a friend's four-year-old said to Cheryl as she piggy-backed him along the beach, "Your hair smells of **strawberries** and **peaches**!" Well, he may not have been accurate on the content, but there cannot be many greater compliments.

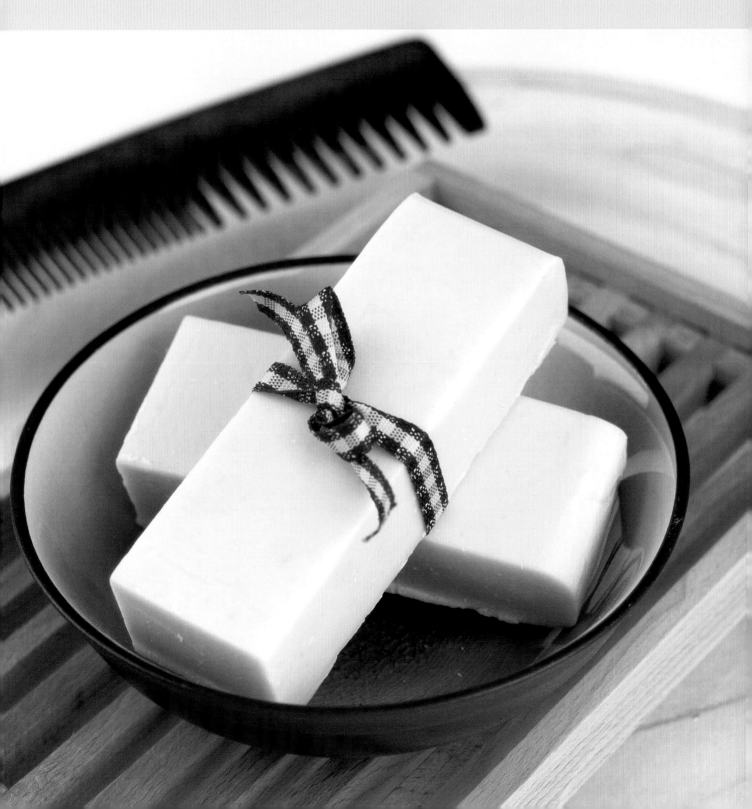

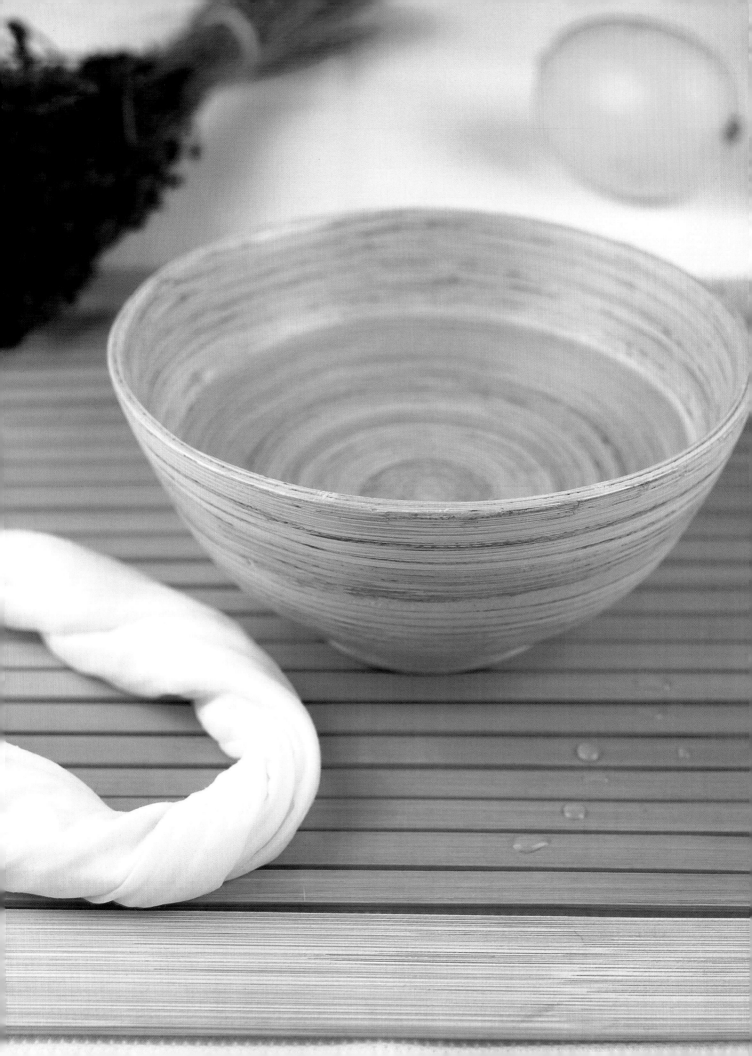

Many headaches are caused by tension. The best way to **relieve** them is to lie down with one pillow under your head and another under your knees, and apply a cold (not icy) essential oil compress to the forehead for 10 minutes. Not only does this help a headache but it is also extremely **soothing** in the case of fever.

The definitive anti-headache essential oil is lavender. Even a drop dabbed on each temple can be **effective**—and just as quick as taking a painkiller. Peppermint is excellent for a "sick" headache, while rosemary and eucalyptus are **perfect** for a "blocked sinus" headache. A combination of lemon and lavender essential oils will also reduce fever.

HEAD-TO-HEAD COMPRESS

Ingredients

Cold water

Essential oils, such as lavender, lemon, peppermint, rosemary, or eucalyptus

Equipment

Large bowl

Clean washcloth

Method

1 Fill a large bowl with cold, but not icy, water. Sprinkle in a couple of drops of essential oil. Swirl a washcloth in the water, then gently wring it out.

2 Place the washcloth over the forehead and leave for 10 minutes. Ideally, you also need an understanding helper to soak and wring the cloth, to refresh it as necessary when it warms up. The combination of relaxation, cooling, and the therapeutic effect of the essential oils will calm and soothe.

Migraines—another story altogether

Migraines, like tension headaches, may well be triggered by stress. However, any sufferer will tell you that the last thing she wanted during an attack is to be near a strong smell, even a lovely essential oil. So for migraine sufferers, prevention is the best form of cure. We suggest using one or more of the recipes featured in the Relax & Rebalance chapter on a regular basis, to keep tension at bay.

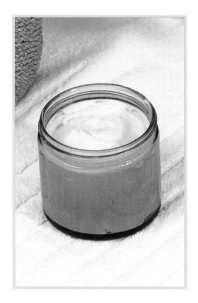

Although often neglected, our feet need a little **tender** loving care, too. Cramped and often hot—and smelly—they deserve a **treat** as good as this lemon and ginger night cream.

Lemon essential oil is an excellent skin conditioner for the tootsies: It treats blisters, tender feet, and brittle nails and generally disinfects and **freshens** the feet. Ginger essential oil will zing circulation and relieve those tired, achy feelings that inevitably result from a hard day.

SOLE-TO-SOLE NIGHT CREAM FOR FEET

Ingredients

½ oz beeswax

½ oz cocoa butter

2 oz coconut oil

2 Tbsp sweet almond oil

4 Tbsp mineral water

1½ tsp lemon essential oil

½ tsp ginger essential oil

Equipment

Stainless-steel saucepan

Wooden spoon

Dark or clear glass jars with lids

Method

1 Place the beeswax, cocoa butter, and coconut and sweet almond oils in a large, heavy-based stainless-steel saucepan and melt over low heat. Add the mineral water in a gentle trickle and beat with a wooden spoon until smooth.

2 Take the saucepan off the heat and keep stirring until the cream has cooled to body temperature. Add the essential oils and mix thoroughly.

3 Decant the cream to airtight jars and shake until the lotion has cooled completely, to stop the oil and water from separating. Store clear glass jars in a dark place to preserve the essential oils.

4 Close to bedtime, take a warm bath, then smooth or gently massage a generous amount of cream into the feet. Put on a pair of cotton socks and allow the treatment to work overnight.

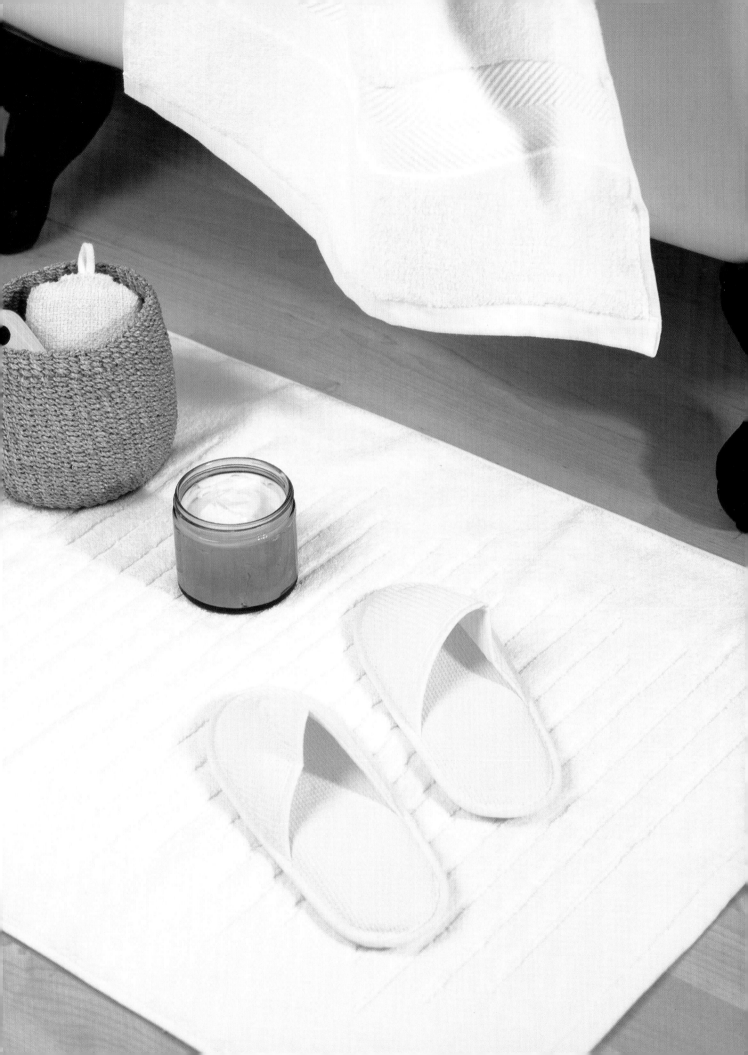

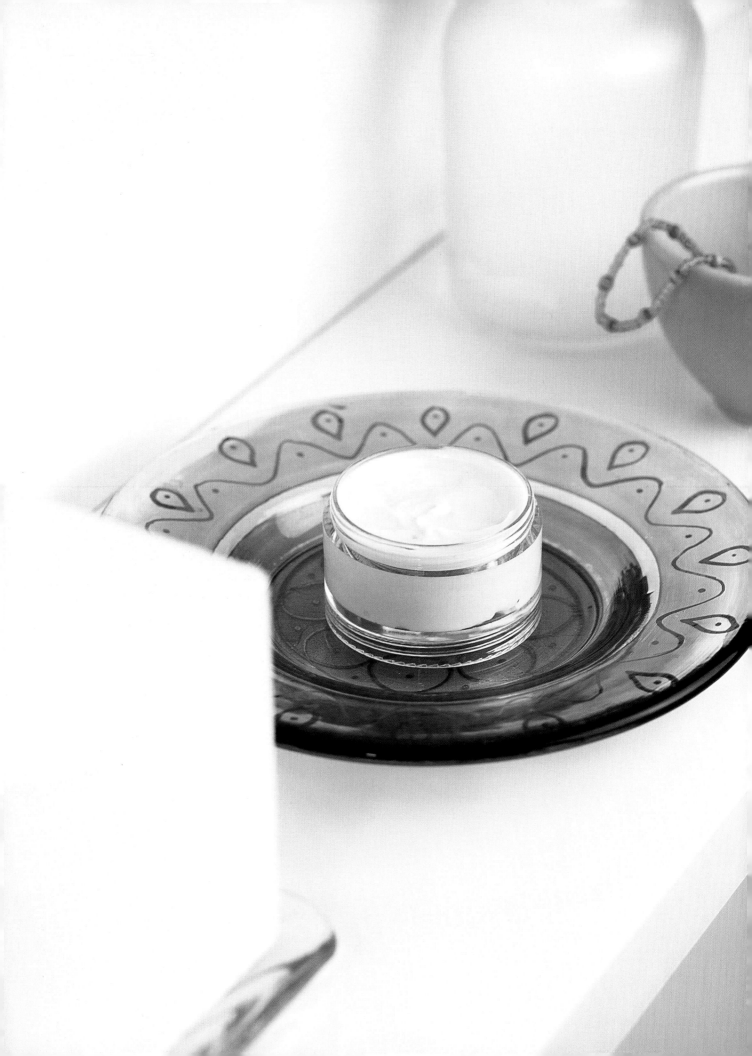

Many of us put our hands through a great deal of abuse: Hard work, cold weather, and harsh detergents all take their toll. Cuts, irritations, brittle and split nails, and dry and cracked skin are common complaints. But help is here courtesy of this **nourishing** cream. Lemon essential oil is invaluable for its antiseptic and anti-aging properties, as well as its mild bleaching effect, useful for stains and liver spots. Lavender will **soothe** even the most irritated skin and stimulate the healing of cuts, cracks, burns, and stings.

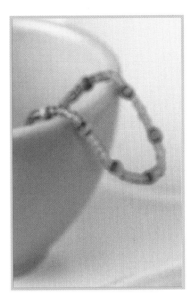

HEALING HANDS NIGHT CREAM

Ingredients

¹/₂ oz beeswax

¹/₂ oz cocoa butter

2 oz coconut oil

2 Tbsp vitamin E oil or wheat germ oil

4 Tbsp mineral water

1 tsp lavender essential oil

1 tsp lemon essential oil

Equipment

Stainless-steel saucepan

Wooden spoon

Dark or clear glass jars with lids

Method

1 Melt the beeswax, cocoa butter, and coconut and vitamin E or wheat germ oils in a large, heavy-based stainless-steel saucepan over low heat. Add the mineral water in a gentle trickle and beat thoroughly with a wooden spoon.

2 Take the saucepan off the heat and keep stirring until the cream has cooled to body temperature. Add the essential oils and mix thoroughly.

3 Decant the cream to airtight jars and shake until the cream has cooled completely, to stop the oil and water from separating. Store clear glass jars in a dark place to protect the mix from light.

4 This rich, nourishing cream is best massaged generously into hands, nails, and cuticles and then left on overnight. Wear pure cotton gloves to aid absorption.

"YOU'RE SO VEIN" VARICOSE VEIN CREAM

Ingredients

7 oz cocoa butter

1 oz coconut oil

³/₄ fl oz calendula oil

2 handfuls of calendula plants: flowers, stems, and leaves

15 drops juniper berry essential oil

15 drops lemon essential oil

Equipment

Stainless-steel saucepan

Wooden spoon

Cotton muslin cloth

Dark or clear glass jars with lids

Method

1 Melt the cocoa butter and coconut and calendula oils in a large, heavy-based stainless-steel saucepan over low heat.

2 Place the calendula plants in the hot oil mixture and stir well with a wooden spoon. It will appear frothy. Remove from the heat, cover, and let sit overnight.

3 The next day, reheat the cream until it melts, then strain it through cotton muslin cloth to remove the calendula plants. Mix in the essential oils. Pour the cream into glass jars and allow to cool completely. Keep clear jars in a dark place to preserve the essential oils.

Avoiding varicose veins

The best advice to avoid the onset of varicose veins is to rest with your legs higher than your heart whenever you have the opportunity, exercise regularly, and avoid standing for extended lengths of time. Don't cross your legs or sit with your feet tucked under you, because this cuts off the circulation. Be careful when massaging varicose veins—don't apply direct pressure and use light stroking movements. Always stroke upward, toward the heart. If in doubt, ask a professional or just smooth the cream gently over the affected areas.

You could also try this calendula tincture. Infuse a small handful of calendula petals in 2 fl oz vodka (see page 20). Cover and leave for 14 days in a warm place, shaking daily. Strain and add 4 fl oz witch hazel. When cool, dab onto the affected areas.

Safety consideration

Do not use juniper berry essential oil while pregnant. Lavender essential oil is a good substitute in this recipe.

Varicose veins are a common problem that affect many men as well as women. Often achy or downright painful, anything that can help to **ease** them is welcome. This gentle cream contains calendula, a **marvelous** plant with many and varied virtues, one of which is that it helps heal skin and remedy varicose veins. Juniper berry essential oil is wonderfully **detoxifying** and helps to alleviate fluid retention, which goes hand in hand with varicose veins and poor circulation. It is also valuable in maintaining the **condition** of the skin.

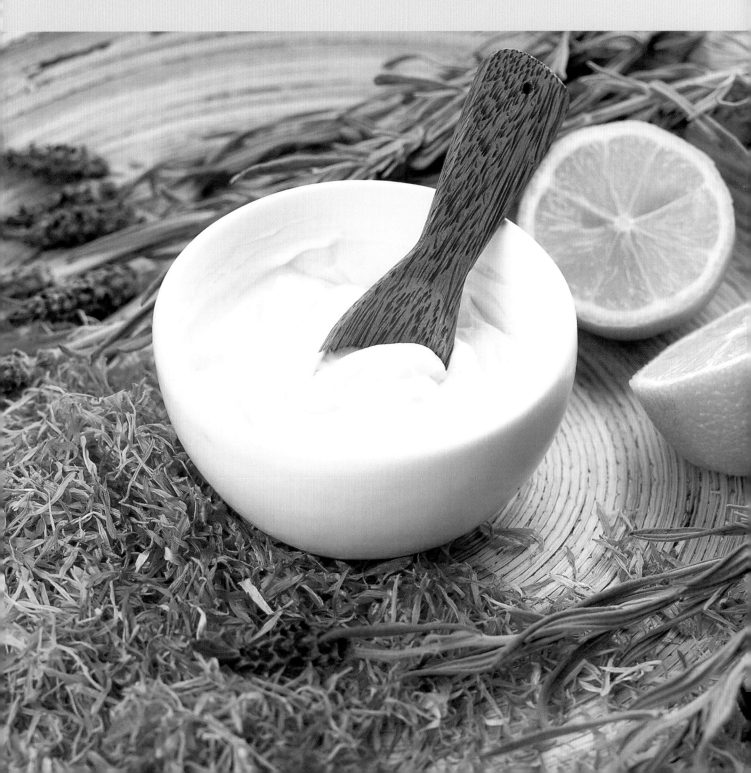

Chamomile essential oil is well known for its soothing, **calming**, and anti-inflammatory qualities. It is used for many skin problems, particularly where there is sensitivity, dryness, and irritation. This includes conditions such as eczema, for which the calming and **stress-relieving** properties are also helpful. We have also added myrrh essential oil to this cream, for its antifungal action. So if you have overdone the gardening or housework, perhaps using too-strong detergents without rubber gloves, try this **soothing** balm.

CHAMOMILE SOOTHER FOR IRRITATED HANDS

Ingredients
2 handfuls of chamomile flowers

9 fl oz water

1 1/2 fl oz sweet almond oil

1 oz beeswax

1 1/2 Tbsp honey

3/4 fl oz wheat germ oil

5 drops Roman chamomile essential oil

5 drops myrrh essential oil

Equipment
Saucepan with lid

Coffee filter paper

Stainless-steel saucepan

Wooden spoon

Dark or clear glass jars with lids

Method

1 Make a chamomile infusion by gently simmering the chamomile flowers in the water in a saucepan with a lid for 30 minutes. Leave covered and allow to cool.

2 Strain through a coffee filter paper to remove flowers; retain liquid.

3 Melt the almond oil and beeswax together in a large, heavy-based stainless-steel saucepan. Add the honey and stir into the mixture with a wooden spoon. Add the wheat germ oil and herbal infusion and beat thoroughly.

4 Take the saucepan off the heat and keep stirring until the cream has cooled to body temperature. Add the essential oils and mix thoroughly, stirring slowly until the cream is cool.

5 Pour the cream into glass jars. Keep clear glass jars in a dark place to preserve the oils.

6 Use this exceptionally rich, superb soothing cream in small quantities, paying special attention to the cuticles.

> ### Safety consideration
> If you are pregnant, substitute lavender oil for the myrrh.

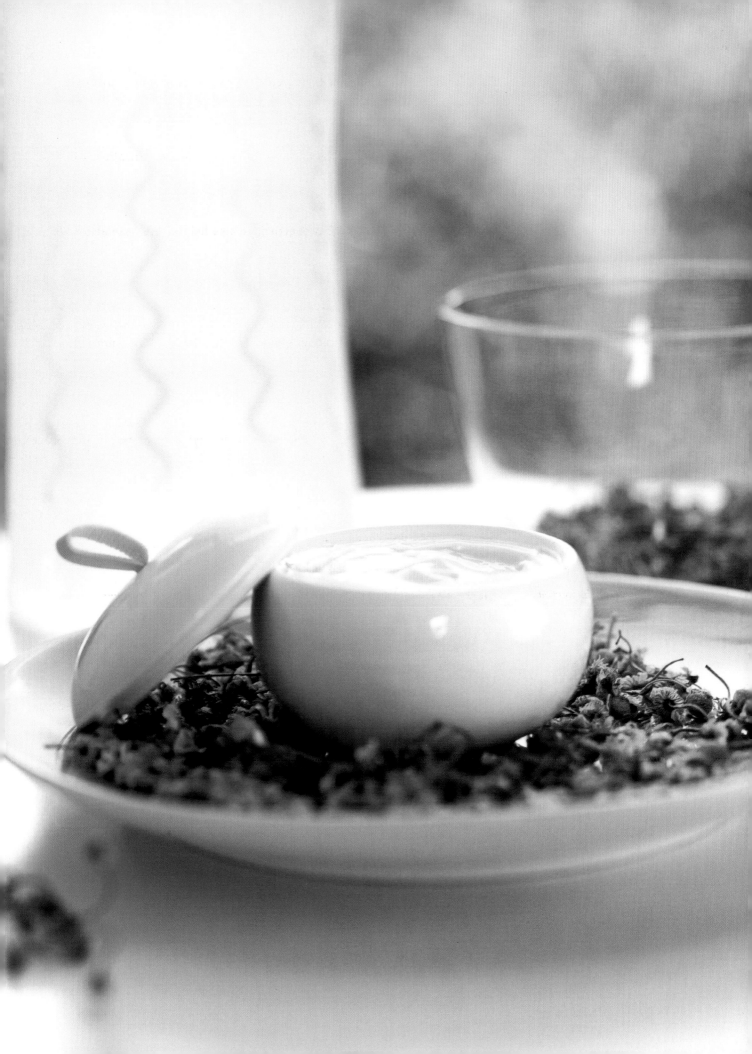

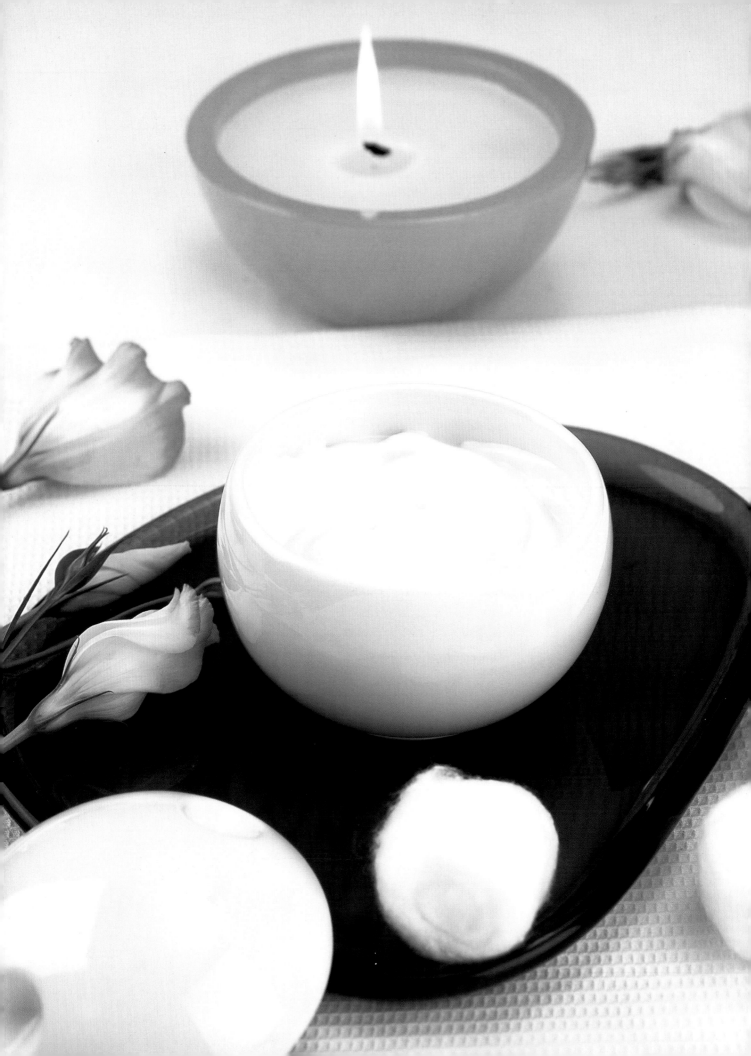

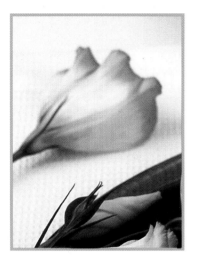

Stretch marks can be an unfortunate legacy of pregnancy. However, we have the antidote! Our cream will soon have you feeling yummy and **glamorous** again. The essential oils of lavender and lemon have a healing effect and reduce the redness of the stretch marks, optimizing the skin's **regenerative** powers. Ylang ylang essential oil is a great skin conditioner and also a powerful aphrodisiac, which will help you to feel **sexy** again.

YUMMY MUMMY STRETCH MARK CREAM

Ingredients

¹/₂ oz beeswax

¹/₂ oz cocoa butter

2 oz coconut oil

2 Tbsp evening primrose oil

4 Tbsp mineral water

1 tsp ylang ylang essential oil

¹/₂ tsp lavender essential oil

¹/₂ tsp lemon essential oil

Equipment

Stainless-steel saucepan

Wooden spoon

Dark or clear glass jars with lids

Method

1 Melt the beeswax, cocoa butter, and the coconut and evening primrose oils in a large, heavy-based stainless-steel saucepan over low heat. Beat in the mineral water with a wooden spoon until you have a smooth mixture.

2 Take the saucepan off the heat and keep stirring until the cream has cooled to body temperature. Add the essential oils and mix thoroughly to make a smooth cream.

3 Decant the cream to airtight jars and shake until the lotion has cooled completely, to stop the oil and water from separating. Store clear glass jars in a dark place to ensure the essential oils are well preserved.

4 Gently smooth the cream into the skin over the offending area. Use daily after a bath or shower and your skin will feel softer after just a few days.

Asian cultures have used hair oils for centuries and know the benefits of head massage to **relax** the large, flat muscles over the scalp: the forehead (where a lot of tension develops) and the base of the skull (the focal point for stress). As well as relaxing the mind and body, the rosemary and lemongrass essential oils will **rejuvenate** your hair, while lavender and geranium essential oils will treat a flaky scalp.

Good **circulation** is all-important for healthy hair. So give your head a real treat, or even better, ask a friend or partner with firm but gentle fingers to massage you. Leave the oil on overnight if you can, wearing a towel turban to protect the pillow. In the A.M., wash with a **gentle** shampoo and dry as normal.

HAIR HEAVEN

Ingredients

4 fl oz sweet almond oil or light olive oil

1/2 tsp geranium essential oil

1/2 tsp lavender essential oil

1/2 tsp lemongrass essential oil

1/2 tsp rosemary essential oil

Equipment

Dark or clear glass bottle with tight-fitting lid

Method

1 Put all the oils in a bottle with a tight lid and shake well. Store clear glass in a dark cupboard, away from little ones.

2 Use before bed. Shake the bottle well, pour about a tablespoon into the palm of your hand, and massage well into the scalp. Wrap head in a towel to protect your pillow and leave overnight. Shampoo out the following morning.

3 Repeat weekly to keep your hair and scalp in good condition.

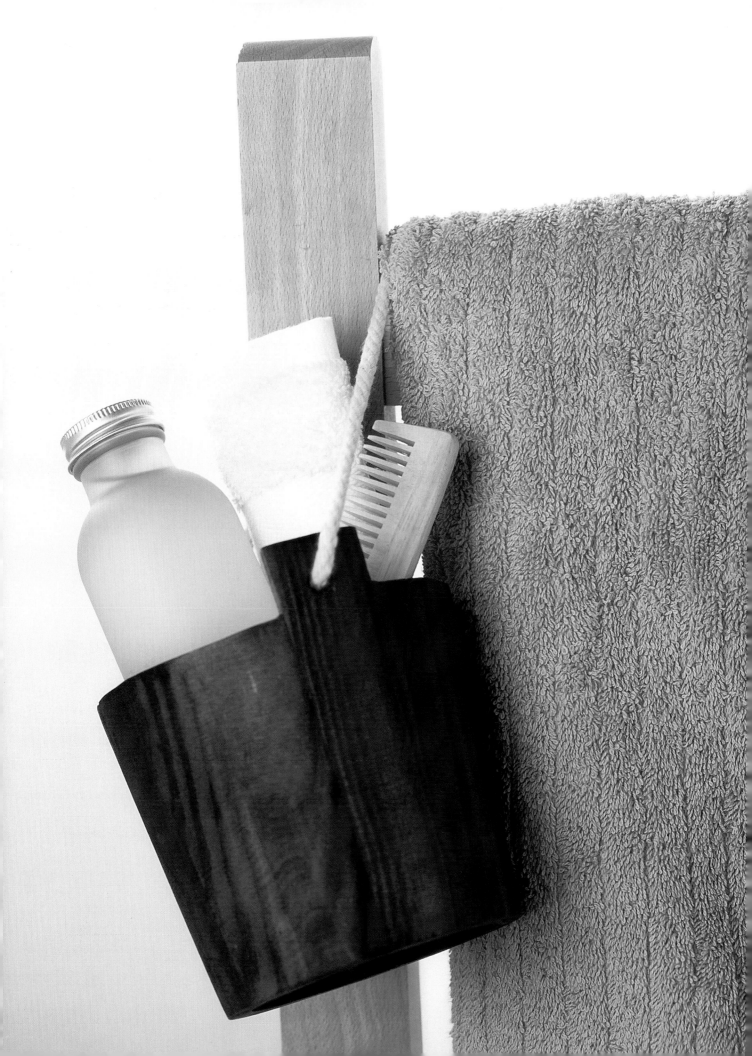

SIX-PACK SOAP

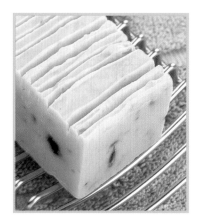

Ingredients

4 fl oz mineral water

2 handfuls of lavatera flowers and stems

A handful of chamomile flowers

4¹/₂ fl oz olive oil

1 oz palm oil

1 oz coconut oil

¹/₂ oz beeswax

1 oz caustic soda

2 tsp bergamot essential oil

1¹/₂ tsp clary sage essential oil

¹/₂ tsp lavender essential oil

¹/₂ tsp patchouli essential oil

Equipment

General equipment (see page 12)

Safety equipment (see page 13)

Method

1. Boil the mineral water with the chamomile and lavatera flowers and stems for two minutes. Allow to cool, then strain, reserving the infusion and flowers. Measure. If shy of 4 fl oz, add more mineral water as necessary.

2. Work in a well-ventilated area. Oil and line a plastic mold with waxed paper.

3. Melt the olive, palm, and coconut oils with the beeswax in a stainless-steel saucepan over low heat.

4. Wearing rubber gloves, an apron, protective eyewear, and a mask, pour the caustic soda into the chamomile and lavatera infusion in a tall plastic bucket. Stir until dissolved with a plastic spatula.

5. Using two jam thermometers, one for the oil and one for the caustic soda mix (lye water), allow both solutions to reach 131°F. Still wearing the protective clothing, immediately pour the lye water into the oil mixture and stir well to thoroughly incorporate the two. Continue to stir well until the mixture traces—when a drizzle leaves a line on the surface of the soap. Pour in the essential oils and a handful of the infused flowers and stir well again.

6. Pour the soap into the prepared mold. Cover with cardboard and leave for 24 hours in a dry, safe, warm place.

7. Remember that the soap is still caustic at this stage, so wear rubber gloves to handle it. Turn it out onto a wooden board covered with waxed paper, remove the lining paper, and cut to the desired sizes with a carving knife. Arrange the soaps on a tray covered with waxed paper and allow to mature for four weeks in a dry, warm place, turning occasionally to assist the drying.

> ### Safety consideration
> Bergamot essential oil makes the skin more sensitive to sunlight, so do not use it before being exposed to the sun.

This is quite a masculine soap, but that is not to say that women won't enjoy using it, too. Clary sage essential oil has a wonderfully **nutty** aroma; it also prevents excessive sweating. Patchouli, with its antiseptic qualities, also acts as a fixative for the other essential oils and gives an **exotic** scent to this soap. Lavender has a list of attributes as long as your arm: In this soap, it balances the other oils. Bergamot blends nicely with these essential oils and prevents sleepiness. It is a cheering, **uplifting** essential oil and adds a lovely citrus top note to the aroma.

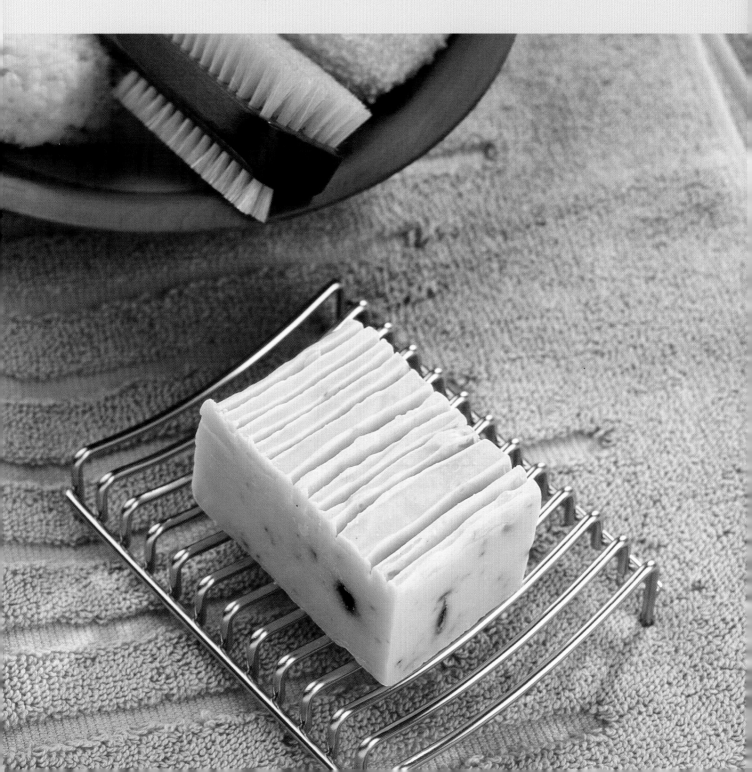

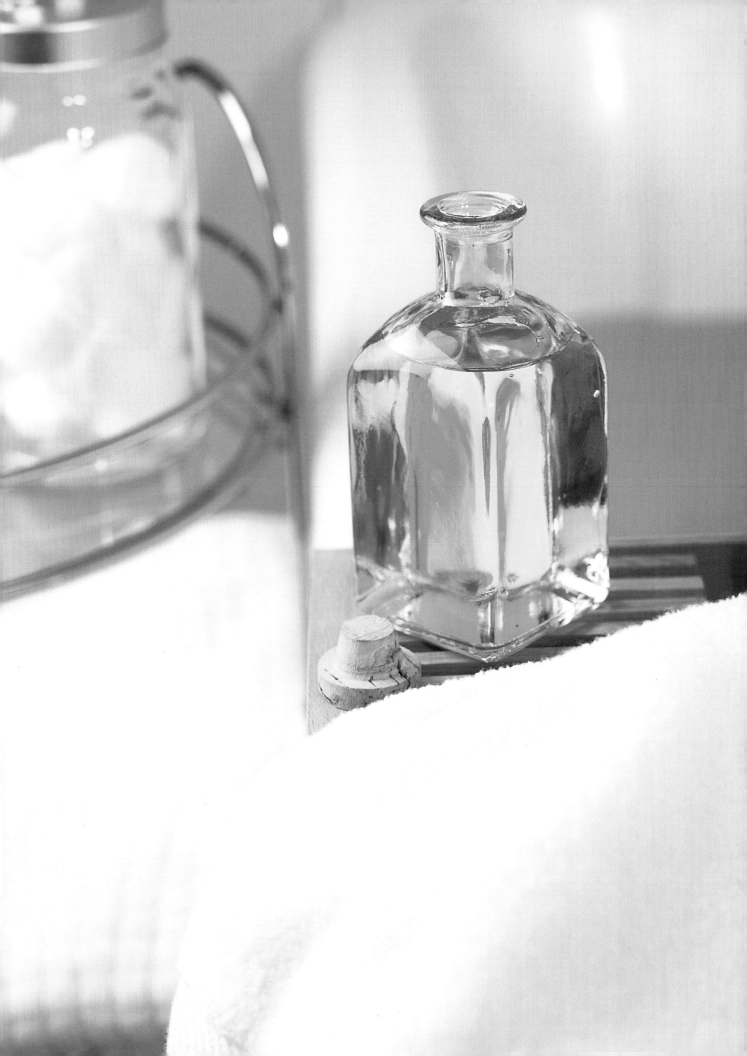

Painful joints will love the feel of a **gentle** rub with this oil. Lavender and rosemary essential oils will ease the aching, while juniper berry oil is well known to improve circulation and **detoxify** the body. Remember that pregnant women should avoid juniper berry essential oil—simply replace with another of your **favorite** oils.

(OH, MY) POOR OLD BONES JOINT OIL

Ingredients

2 fl oz sweet almond oil

6 drops lavender essential oil

4 drops juniper berry essential oil

2 drops rosemary essential oil

Equipment

Dark or clear glass bottle with tight-fitting lid

Method

1 Mix all the ingredients together in a bottle with a tight-fitting lid. Store a clear glass bottle in a dark place to preserve the essential oils.

2 Warmth is a great relief for arthritic joints, so rub this in after a warm bath for maximum effect, then wear something loose, such as a sweatsuit or pajamas, and relax with your body well supported.

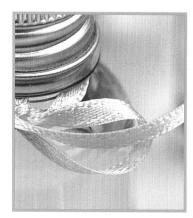

This is a wonderfully balancing facial oil for all skin types. Rosehip oil is the finest base oil for **delicate** skin and is readily absorbed with no greasiness. Geranium essential oil balances sebum production and **nourishes** dry or combination skins. Ylang ylang is the most feminine of all essential oils and, like geranium, it **balances** the complexion, making it suitable for dry or combination skins.

FABULOUS FACIAL OIL

Ingredients

4 fl oz rosehip oil

10 drops ylang ylang essential oil

4 drops geranium essential oil

Equipment

Dark or clear glass bottle with tight-fitting lid

Method

1 Place all the ingredients in a bottle and shake gently to combine. If you are using a clear glass bottle, store in a dark place to preserve the essential oils.

2 Use this oil nightly, before going to bed, to allow the oil to fully absorb into your skin while you sleep for an ultraconditioning effect. Apply to warm, thoroughly cleansed skin.

Rosehips

Rosehip oil is a natural preservative that also eases inflammation. Rosehips have other uses, too—long before the discovery of vitamin C, rosehip tea was taken to combat the common cold.

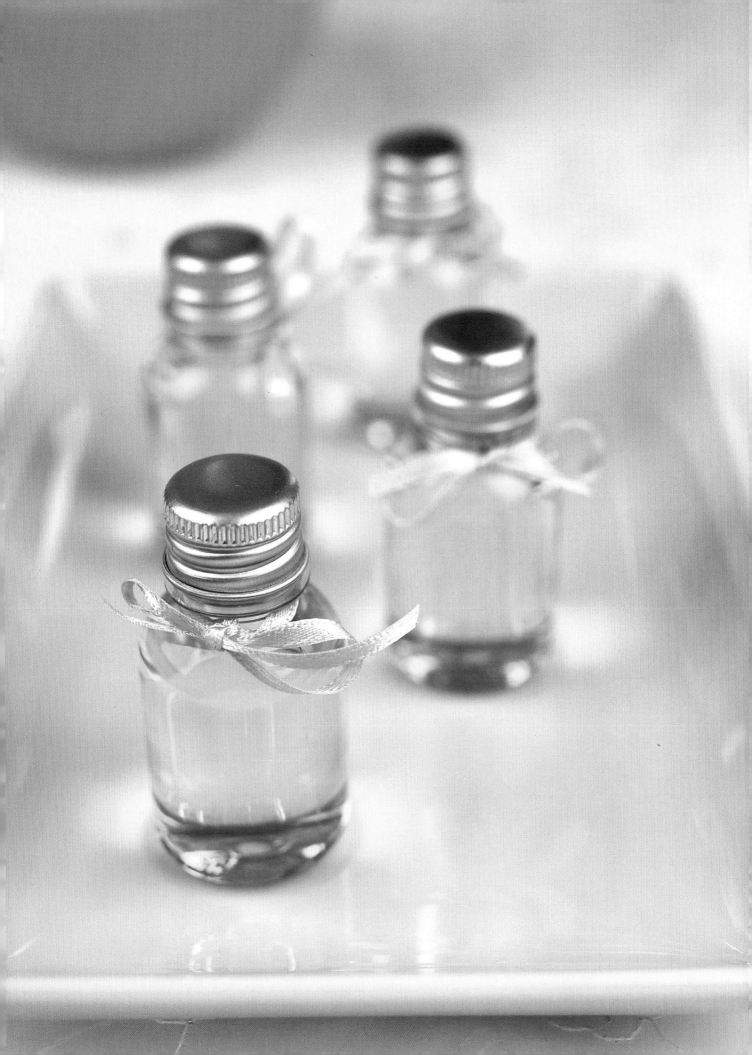

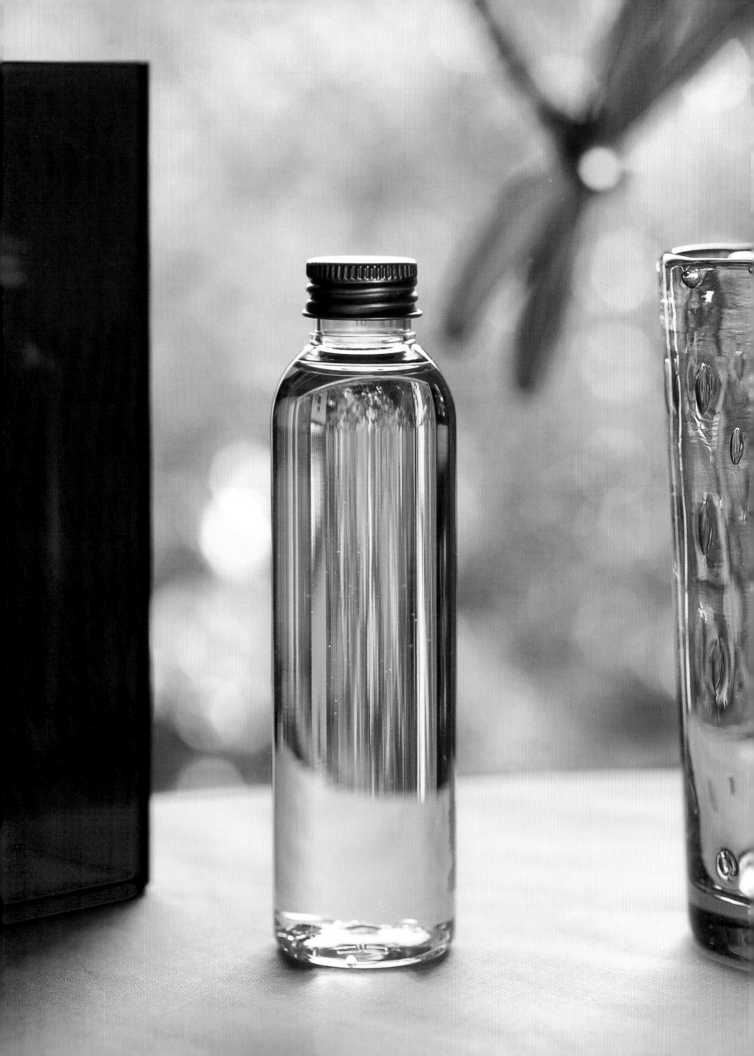

At some time we all get too much sun and are left feeling pink and sore. When that happens, use this oil to calm and soothe both you and your skin. Lavender essential oil has powerful healing properties, having been proved effective in treating even severe burns. It is antiseptic and will calm the inflammation and ease the pain associated with sunburn. Chamomile essential oil also soothes the inflammation and has a calming effect on the body, promoting relaxation and restful sleep.

"WHAT A SCORCHER" SUNBURN OIL

Ingredients

2 Tbsp sweet almond oil

6 drops lavender essential oil

2 drops Roman chamomile essential oil

Equipment

Dark or clear glass bottle with tight-fitting lid

Method

1 Place all the ingredients in a bottle with a tight-fitting lid and shake well. Store clear glass in a dark place to preserve the essential oils.

2 If you can't bear to smooth the oil directly onto your skin, a few drops of the mixture run into a tepid bath is of great relief. Pat dry with a soft towel and wear soft, loose clothes to avoid rubbing the skin.

Traditional sunburn remedy

If you don't have the ingredients for this recipe handy, try mixing two teaspoons of tomato juice and four tablespoons of buttermilk and applying to the affected area. Leave for half an hour, then wash off.

GIFTWRAPPING IDEAS

The natural look is perfect for wrapping some of the healing products from this chapter—and comes

across as very smart. Wooden or cardboard boxes can be filled with shredded tissue or raffia, while a

bundle of cinnamon sticks or a slice of dried fruit adds a special touch. Skeleton leaves or

pieces of bark can be wrapped

around a soap and tied with raffia.

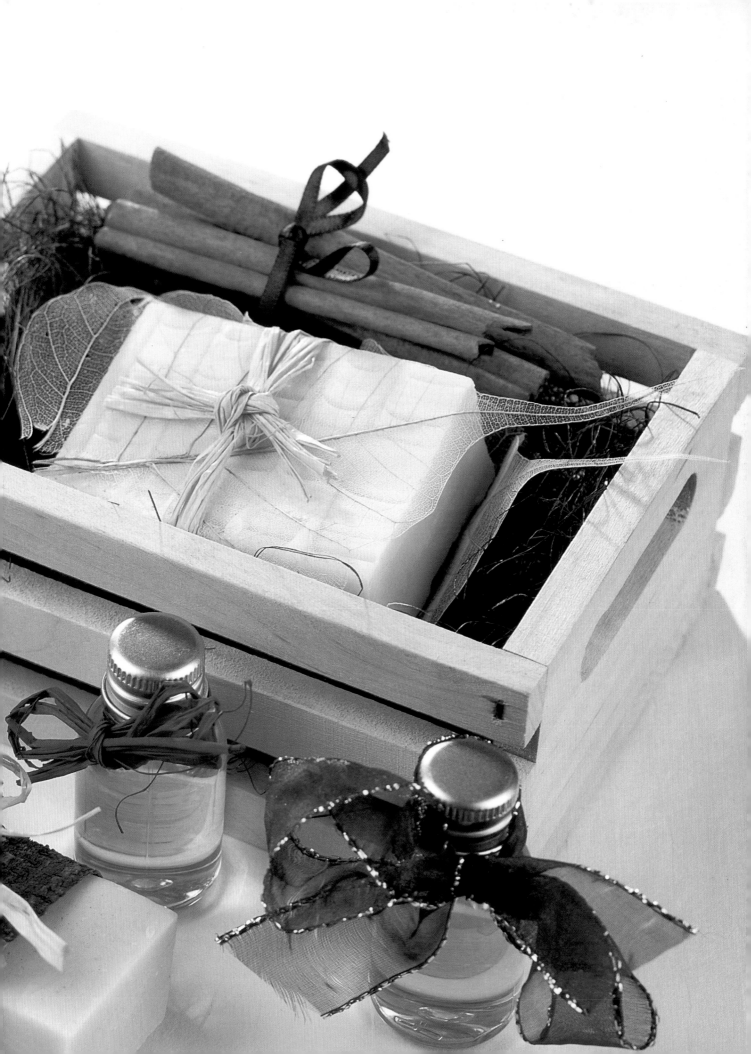

SUPPLIERS & USEFUL ADDRESSES

UNITED STATES

Bramble Berry
Otion: The Soap Bar (retail location)
1427 Railroad Avenue
Bellingham, WA 98225
Tel: (360) 676-1030
www.brambleberry.com
Supplies bases, essential oils, dried herbs and flowers, molds, and soapmaking equipment. Online shopping service available.

Camden-Grey Essential Oils
3591 NW 82 Avenue
Miami, FL 33122
Tel: (305) 500-9630
Email: orderdesk
@camdengrey.com
www.camdengrey.com
Stocks bases, essential oils, dried herbs, molds, and glassware. Online shopping service available.

Essential Wholesale
8850 SE Herbert Court
Clackamas, OR 97015
Tel: (503) 722-7557
Email: info
@essentialwholesale.com
www.essentialwholesale.com
Stocks soapmaking raw materials, oils, and molds.

From Nature With Love
P.O. Box 201
Hawleyville, CT 06440
Tel: (203) 267-6061
Email: information
@fromnaturewithlove.com
www.fromnaturewithlove.com
Supplies soapmaking raw materials, oils, dried herbs and flowers, equipment, packaging, molds, and cutters.

Soap Crafters
2944 S. West Temple
Salt Lake City, UT 84115
Tel: (801) 484-5121
Email: emails
@soapcrafters.com
www.soapcrafters.com
Supplies soapmaking raw materials, oils, dried herbs and flowers, bottles and jars, and equipment.

SunFeather Natural Soap Company
1551 Highway 72
Potsdam, NY 13676
Tel: (315) 265-3648
Email: sunsoap@sunsoap.com
www.sunsoap.com
Stocks soapmaking raw materials, supplies and utensils, oils, and molds.

UNITED KINGDOM

Essentially Oils
8–10 Mount Farm
Junction Road
Churchill
Chipping Norton
Oxfordshire OX7 6NP
Tel: (01608) 659544
Email: sales@essentiallyoils.com
www.essentiallyoils.com
Supplies essential oils, carrier oils, bottles, jars, and other soapmaking essentials.

Holland & Barrett
Samuel Ryder House
Townsend Drive
Attleborough Fields
Nuneaton
Warwickshire CV11 6XW
Tel: (0870) 606 6606
www.hollandandbarrett.com
Stores throughout the UK sell essential oils and dried herbs and flowers. Online shopping service available.

Meadows Aromatherapy Products
Park Farm Oast
Canterbury Road
Boughton Aluph
Ashford
Kent TN25 4EW
Tel: (0845) 060 0123
Email: enquiries
@meadowsaroma.com
www.meadowsaroma.com
Supplies essential oils, base oils, and soapmaking products.

Neals Yard Remedies
15 Neals Yard
Covent Garden
London WC2H 9DP
Tel: (020) 7379 7222
www.nealsyardremedies.co.uk
Supplies oils, essential oils, bottles and jars, plus herbs and dried flowers. Branches

throughout the UK. Online shopping service available.

William Hodgson & Co
73a London Road
Alderley Edge
Cheshire SK9 7DY
Tel: (01625) 599111
Supplies base oils, including coconut, palm, and vegetable oils (minimum 1 kilo quantity).

SOUTH AFRICA

Aromatic Aromatherapy
Victoria & Alfred Waterfront
Waterfront
Cape Town 8000
Tel: (021) 418 0648
Supplies essential oils.

Cagey Bee
Shop 3, 1 Olifants Road
Emmerentia 2195
Tel: (011) 888 6583
Email: hansh@metroweb.co.za
Stocks soapmaking products, molds, etc.

Moco Cosmetic Packaging
18 Auret Street
Jeppestown 2094
Tel: (011) 624 3493/4
Email: moco@absamail.co.za
Supplies high-quality glass and plastic bottles and jars.

Parsons Home Appliances
46 Market Square
Kimberley 8301
Tel: (053) 832 9404/5/6/7
Email: info@parsons.co.za
www.parsons.co.za
Stocks soapmaking products and soap molds.

AUSTRALIA

AquaSapone
110 Translator Rd, Armidale
NSW 2350
Tel: (02) 6772 0300
www.aquasapone.com.au
Supplies soapmaking products, molds and essential oils.

Aussie Soap Supplies
Tel: (08) 9339 1885
Email: heyjude@iinet.com.au
www.aussiesoapsupplies.com.au
Supplies soapmaking raw materials, oils, and containers.

Australian Botanical Products
36 Meleveton Drive
Hallam Vic 3803
Tel: (03) 9796 4833
www.essentialoils.com.au
Stocks aromatherapy oils, soapmaking products, and a range of containers.

Heirloom Body Care
78 Barnes Road
Llandilo
NSW 2747
Tel: (02) 4777 4457
Email: heirloom
   @heirloombodycare.com.au
www.heirloombodycare.com.au
Supplies soapmaking raw materials, oils, fragrances, and glassware.

Luscious Skin Care
19 Belltrees Close,
Glen Alpine
NSW 2560
Tel: (02) 4626 7822
Email: info
   @lusciousskincare.com

www.lusciousskincare.com.au
Supplies carrier and essential oils, bottles, and jars.

NEW ZEALAND

Aromatherapy New Zealand Ltd
PO Box 47 470
Ponsonby
Auckland
Tel: (64) 523 5969
www.aroma.co.nz
Supplies a wide range of essential oils.

Aromatics & More Ltd
9 Trading Place
Henderson
PO Box 37
Waitakere, Auckland
Tel: (64) 9 835 4330
www.aromaticsandmore.com
Supplies soapmaking supplies, essential oils, fragrances, and packaging materials.

FURTHER READING AND USEFUL WEBSITES

The Practice of Aromatherapy,
   Dr Jean Valnet,
   The CW Daniel Company Ltd

Aromatherapy: An A-Z
   Patricia David
   The CW Daniel Company Ltd

www.thesoapopera.co.uk

www.thesoapkitchen.co.uk

INDEX